99
bath time treats

First edition for the United States and Canada published by Barron's Educational Series, Inc., 2005

First published in the UK by: MQ Publications Limited
12 The Ivories,
6-8 Northampton Street,
London N1 2HY
www.mqpublications.com

Copyright © MQ Publications Limited 2005
Text copyright © Susannah Marriott 2005
Design by Balley Design Associates
This Translation of 99 Bath Time Treats is published by arrangement with MQ Publications Limited

Library of Congress Catalog Card No.:
2004104912
International Standard Book No.:
0-7641-5810-4

Printed and bound in China

This book contains the opinions and ideas of the author. It is intended to provide helpful and informative material on the subjects addressed in this book and is sold with the understanding that the author and publisher are not engaged in rendering medical, health, or any other kind of personal professional services in this book. The reader should consult his or her medical, health, or other competent professional before adopting any of the suggestions in this book or drawing references form it. The author and publisher disclaim all responsibility for any liability, loss, or risk, personal or otherwise, which is incurred as a consequence, directly or indirectly, of the use and application of any of the contents of this book.

9 8 7 6 5 4 3 2 1

Acknowledgments

Thanks to Caudalie, and to Kim Collier at Jamu Spa for kindly providing the winter healing bath and banana face clay recipes.

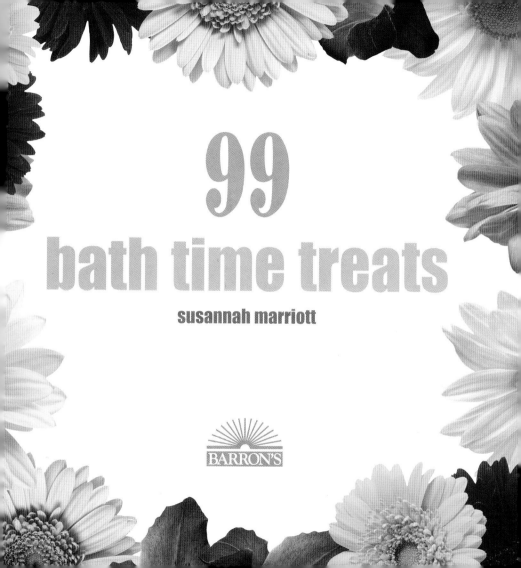

99
bath time treats

susannah marriott

BARRON'S

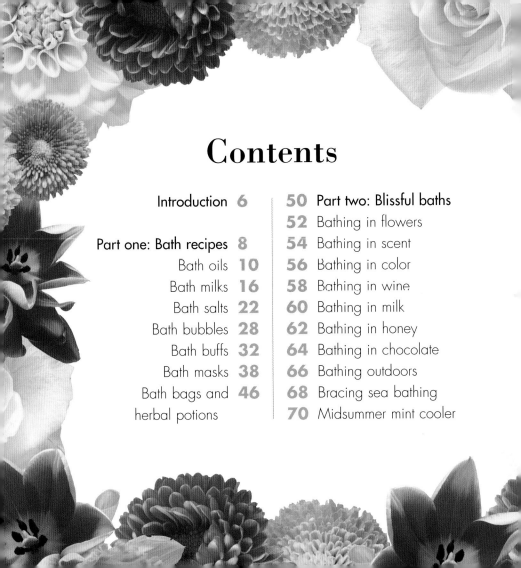

Contents

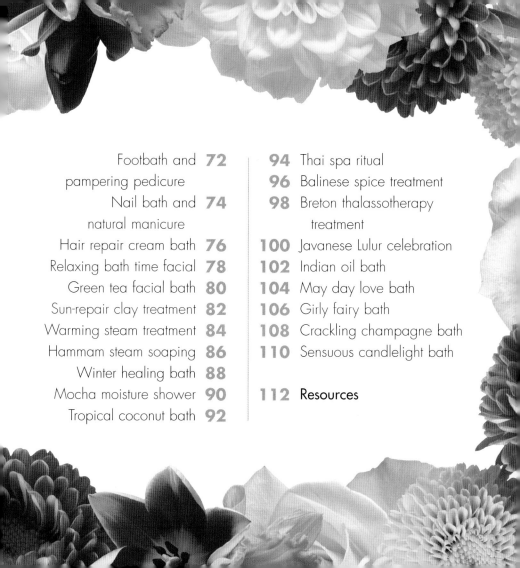

introduction

Wash away your troubles and ease your aching bones by wallowing in a luxurious bath. While you're there, smear on a face mask, apply hot conditioning oils to your hair, paint your nails, or do nothing more strenuous than flip through a magazine or sip a flute of chilled champagne. Be reassured that all the bath products in this book are clean and green. They are often made from food-grade ingredients you might find in your kitchen cupboard and refrigerator: honey and cream, almonds and coconut, chocolate and cinnamon. Not only are they a treat to tempt the palate—some of the masks could double up as dessert—they are free from the harsh detergents and gasoline derivatives that fill off-the-shelf beauty products and have been linked with health concerns. Some of these bathing treatments can be performed at lunchtime; others take all evening. When your skin looks pale, gray, and flaky, and you just can't lift yourself from the couch, let these transformative treats brighten your complexion, lift your spirits, restore your *joie de vivre*, and relax every part of you. Just don't plan to do anything afterward that requires brainpower!

Cautions

If you have health concerns, consult your doctor before using bath treatments, and read the following contraindications:

Hot baths: Avoid very hot baths during pregnancy, and if you have high blood pressure, heart or vascular disease, or varicose veins.

Steam treatments: Avoid if you have asthma, respiratory, or heart conditions.

Salts and seaweed: Do not use Epsom, mineral, or sea salts if you are pregnant or have high blood pressure or heart disease; avoid seaweed if you are allergic to seafood or iodine or if taking thyroxine.

Scrubs and masks: Avoid whole-body exfoliation and body masks if you have blood pressure or heart problems, while you are ill or recovering from illness, and during pregnancy. Avoid nut-based preparations if you are allergic to nuts.

Essential oils: Use only the oils specified, and never use more drops than recommended. Omit those oils suggested if pregnant or breast-feeding, and if you have high blood pressure, kidney problems, or epilepsy. Some citrus oils cause photosensitivity after use when skin is exposed to sunlight, leading to permanent brown patches on the skin. See cautions on individual treatments, omitting citrus oils if you plan to be outdoors or use a sunlamp in the 6 hours following use. If you have any doubts, omit essential oils altogether.

Massage: Avoid if you have a fever, high blood pressure, or skin problems. If you have any other health condition, consult your doctor before massage.

part one
Bath recipes

These are home-spa recipes for supersoft skin and inner glow: silky oils and milks to scent the water in your tub, face masks and body scrubs to deep cleanse your skin and make it sparkle, massage oil blends and dusting powders to anoint a luxuriously bath-softened body. Choose from the soporific and the stimulating, the firming and the toning, the preening and the polishing, mixing custom-made bath blends to match your mood and skin type. All the recipes are easy to make using ingredients you might find in your kitchen—and yes, some of them *are* good enough to eat. Raid your garden for rose petals, get your mixing bowl out, and start running that bath now.

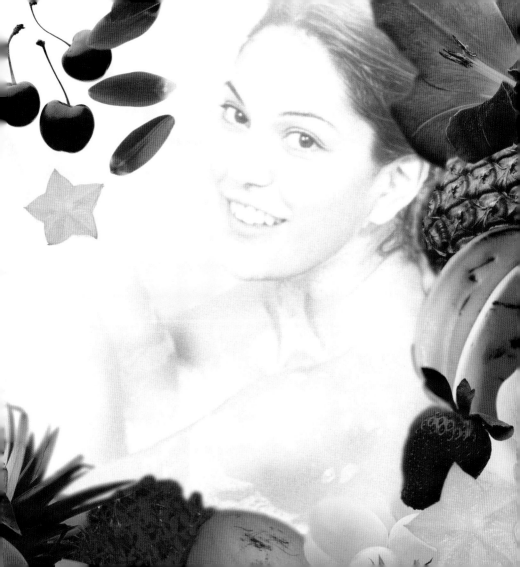

Bath oils

Pouring a little oil into the bathtub creates a silky textured bathwater that's heavenly to sink into and that leaves the skin with a smooth sheen. When you add essential oils to the blend, you surround yourself with exquisite fragrances that can pep you up or relax mind and muscles, according to the blend you select. Extracted from flowers and leaves, fruit and berries, bark and resins, essential oils are the highly concentrated essence of a plant, and almost always need to be diluted in a "base" or "carrier" oil. In the steamy environment of a bathroom these oils release their potent molecules readily, and skin softened by hot water absorbs oils efficiently, so never use more drops than recommended—and don't be tempted to add extra once the initial scent "wears off" (see also cautions on page 7). Experiment with the combinations suggested on these pages until you find a mix that suits you. Then make that your signature bath scent of the season.

Patch testing: If you have very sensitive skin, always do a patch test before using any essential oils: blend 2 drops of the oil you plan to use in 1 tsp sweet almond oil. Dab the mixture on the inside of your elbow. Wait 12 hours; if you notice a reaction such as redness or itching, avoid this oil. To remedy skin reactions, soothe the affected area with more sweet almond oil, then rinse it under cold running water.

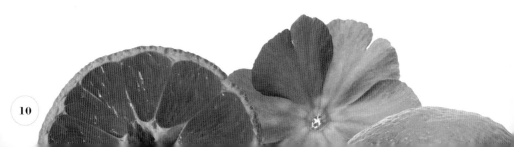

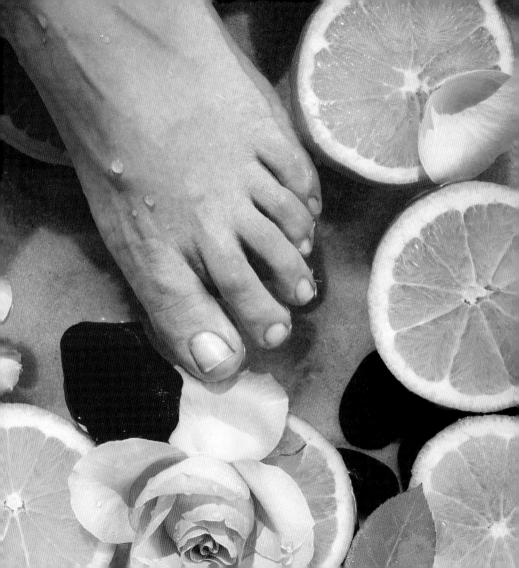

1. JASMINE SKINCARE OIL

Ingredients

4 tbsp sweet almond oil | 8 drops essential oil of jasmine

Blend the oils to use for body massage, or mix only 1 tsp sweet almond oil with the oil of jasmine to pour into the bath, swishing to disperse just before stepping in. For extra skincare, spoon into the bath 2 tbsp orange blossom water. Avoid during pregnancy.

2. MALAY SPICE BATH OIL

Ingredients

1 tsp sweet almond oil | 2 drops each essential oils of orange,
1 drop essential oil of ginger | ylang ylang, and patchouli

Mix the oils together and swish into the bath before climbing in. Avoid sunlight and sunlamps for 6 hours after use. If you have sensitive skin, do a patch test for ginger oil.

3. JOYFUL SCENT BATH OIL

Ingredients

1 tsp sweet almond oil | 3 drops each essential oils of ylang
| ylang, frankincense, and jasmine

Blend all the oils then swish into the bathtub before stepping in. Omit jasmine oil during pregnancy. If you have sensitive skin, do a patch test for ylang ylang oil.

4 EASTERN MOISTURE BALM

Ingredients

3 tbsp sweet almond oil
2 tsp wheatgerm oil
1 vitamin E capsule

3 drops each essential oils of jasmine, sandalwood, and patchouli

Blend the oils to use for body massage, or make up the balm with only 1 tsp sweet almond oil to pour into the bath just before stepping in. Blend the almond and wheatgerm oils, then prick the vitamin E capsule and squeeze in the contents. Drop in the essential oils. Omit jasmine oil during pregnancy.

5 WINE BATH OIL

Ingredients

1 tsp grapeseed oil
3 drops each essential oils of rose and lavender

2 drops essential oil of mandarin
1 drop each essential oils of pine and basil

Blend all the oils, then swish into the bathtub just before stepping in. During pregnancy use only mandarin oil. Avoid sunlight and sunlamps for 6 hours after use.

Bathtime massage blends

6   COCONUT HAIR-CONDITIONING OIL

Into 1 tbsp coconut oil and 1 tbsp avocado oil add 3 drops essential oil of ylang ylang and 2 drops lavender. Omit lavender oil during the first trimester of pregnancy; if you have sensitive skin, do a patch test for ylang ylang oil.

7   SKIN-CLEANSING OIL

Into 1 ½ tbsp sweet almond oil squeeze the contents of 1 vitamin E capsule. Add 3 drops each essential oils of neroli and chamomile, 1 drop benzoin. Pour into the bath or use a little on a cotton ball to cleanse the face. Omit chamomile in the first trimester of pregnancy.

8   FACIAL MASSAGE BLEND

Into 2 tbsp sweet almond oil add 2 drops each essential oils of rose and frankincense for mature skin; 2 drops each chamomile and jasmine for sensitive skin; 2 drops each neroli and rose for dry skin; 2 drops each lavender and geranium for oily skin; 4 drops frankincense during pregnancy.

9   INDIAN FACE BALM

Into 1 tbsp peach-kernel oil and 1 tbsp wheatgerm oil add 3 drops essential oil of jasmine and 1 drop basil. Avoid during pregnancy; if you have sensitive skin, do a patch test for basil oil.

10   INDIAN BODY BLEND

Into 4 tbsp sesame seed oil mix 4 drops essential oil of pine, 2 drops each basil and coriander, 1 drop cardamom. Omit basil during pregnancy; if you have sensitive skin, do a patch test for basil, cardamom, and pine oils.

TURKISH MASSAGE BLEND

Into 4 tbsp sweet almond oil blend 8 drops essential oil of lavender and 2 drops each melissa and eucalyptus. Omit eucalyptus if you have high blood pressure or epilepsy, melissa during pregnancy, lavender in the first trimester.

COOLING MASSAGE OIL

Into 2 tbsp sunflower oil stir 2 tbsp aloe vera gel until combined. Then add 8 drops essential oil of lavender, 4 drops tea tree oil, 2 drops oil of geranium. Omit essential oil of geranium during pregnancy, lavender in the first trimester. If you have sensitive skin, do a patch test for tea tree oil.

ANTICELLULITE MASSAGE BLEND

Into 2 tbsp sesame seed oil blend 3 drops each essential oils of rosemary and lavender and 2 drops juniper. Avoid during pregnancy. If you have high blood pressure or epilepsy omit rosemary.

LEMON AND GINGER FOOT MASSAGE OIL

Into 2 tbsp olive oil blend 2 drops each essential oils of ginger and lemon. If you have sensitive skin, do a patch test for the essential oils.

PEPPERMINT FOOT CREAM

Melt ½ oz (15 g) beeswax in a bowl over a pan of boiling water, stirring continuously. Remove from the heat and stir in 6 tbsp olive oil and 12 drops essential oil of peppermint. Keep stirring until cool, spoon into a sterilized dark glass jar, cover with a lid, and refrigerate. Avoid while pregnant or breast-feeding. If you have sensitive skin, do a patch test for peppermint oil.

Bath milks

Act like Cleopatra with these indulgent bathtime concoctions of milk, honey, highly scented essential oils, spices, and herbs. Applied to the skin, milk, cream, and yogurt have soothing properties and especially suit sensitive complexions. The lactic acid in dairy produce is an alphahydroxy acid, an effective natural exfoliator. Beauty therapists also rate dairy products for imparting nutrients, including vitamins A and D, that are vital for maintaining youthful-looking skin. Either pour a pint of organic whole milk into your bath—nothing else feels quite so extravagant—or use these powdered milk base options. Once you find a combination you like, make up enough for a few baths and store in sterilized dark glass containers with tight covers in a cool dark place for a week or so. For the lactose intolerant, we include a luxuriously tropical-scented coconut milk bath.

Caution: Avoid cow milk baths if you are allergic to dairy products. Substitute with goat or sheep milk alternatives, if tolerated.

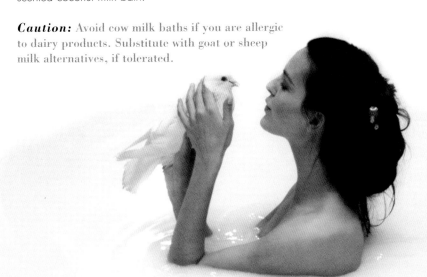

APHRODISIAC MILK BATH

Ingredients

12 tbsp powdered milk | 4 drops essential oil of patchouli
6 drops essential oil of jasmine |

Place the powdered milk in a large bowl and dilute with double the amount of
cool water, adding the liquid gradually and stirring to prevent lumps.
Drop in the essential oils and pour into the bath as it runs.
Omit jasmine oil during pregnancy.

JASMINE MILK BATH

Ingredients

12 tbsp powdered milk | 2 drops essential oil of neroli
2 tbsp rosewater | handfuls of petals: look for rose, orange
6 drops essential oil of jasmine | blossom, and jasmine

Place the powdered milk in a large bowl and dilute with double the amount of
cool water, adding the liquid gradually and stirring to prevent lumps. Stir in the
rosewater. Drop in the essential oils and pour into the bath as it runs, strewing
the petals over the surface of the water. Place a strainer over the drain when
emptying the bath. Omit jasmine oil during pregnancy.

18   COCONUT MILK BATH

Ingredients

1 small can coconut milk	2 drops each essential oils of lemongrass
½ lime, freshly sliced	and vetivert

As the bath runs, pour in the coconut milk and throw the lime slices into the water. After turning off the faucet and before stepping into the tub, drop in the essential oils, swishing to disperse.

19   CHOCOLATE VANILLA MILK BATH

Ingredients

2 vanilla pods	2 tbsp cocoa powder
8 tbsp powdered milk	1 tbsp cornstarch

Throw the vanilla pods into the water as the bath fills. In a large bowl, mix together the powdered milk, cocoa, and cornstarch. Add enough cold water to make a runny paste, adding the liquid little by little and stirring constantly to prevent lumps. Pour into the bathtub as the faucet runs. After the bath collect the vanilla pods, rinse, dry, and set aside for another bath.

20   MILK AND HONEY SOAK

Ingredients

4 tbsp thin honey | 1 tsp avocado oil
8 tbsp powdered milk | 6 drops essential oil of lavender

In a large bowl, stir the honey into the powdered milk to make a thick paste. Moisten with the avocado oil, then dilute with a cup of boiling water, stirring well to eliminate lumps. Pour into the water as you fill the tub. Omit lavender oil during the first trimester of pregnancy.

21   MILK AND ROSE PETAL BATH BAG

Ingredients

handful dried rose petals | 6 drops essential oil of rose
12 tbsp powdered milk |

Pound the rose petals using a pestle and mortar until they are reduced to dust. Place the powdered milk and rose petals in the center of a large square of muslin, drop on the essential oil, and tie to secure. Suspend beneath the hot faucet while the bath runs, or float it in the water. Omit rose oil during pregnancy.

SPICED MILK BATH

Ingredients

10 tbsp powdered milk	2 drops essential oil of coriander
1 cinnamon stick, broken in two	1 drop essential oil of ginger
2 vanilla pods	

In a wide mixing bowl, mix together the powdered milk with enough cold water to make a smooth paste, adding the liquid little by little and stirring constantly to prevent lumps. Pour into the bath as it runs, then throw in the cinnamon pieces and vanilla pods. Just before stepping into the tub, drop in the essential oils and swish to disperse. After the bath, collect the vanilla pods, rinse, dry, and set aside for another bath.

CITRUS MILK BATH

Ingredients

12 tbsp powdered milk	½ lime
½ orange	½ lemon

In a wide mixing bowl, mix together the milk powder with enough cold water to make a smooth paste, adding the liquid little by little and stirring constantly to prevent lumps. Pour into the bath as it runs. Slice the fruit and throw into the bath (place a strainer over the drain when emptying the bath).

24   LEMONGRASS MILK BATH BAG

Ingredients

12 tbsp powdered milk | 6 drops essential oil of geranium
2 sticks of lemongrass, cut into
1-inch-long chunks

Pile the powdered milk and lemongrass in the center of a large square of muslin, drop on the essential oil, and tie to secure. Suspend beneath the hot faucet while the bath is running, or float it in the water. Omit geranium oil during pregnancy.

25   EGYPTIAN MILK BATH

Ingredients

12 tbsp powdered milk | 3 drops each essential oils of
2 tsp ground cinnamon | frankincense, myrrh, and cypress

In a large bowl, mix together the powdered milk and cinnamon. Stir in enough cold water to make a smooth paste, adding the liquid little by little and stirring constantly to prevent lumps. Drop in the essential oils. Pour into the bath, swishing to disperse, just before stepping in. Omit myrrh and cypress oils during pregnancy.

Bath salts

Hot baths scattered with sea and mineral salts help revive tired skin and relieve aches and pains. They also have a detoxifying action, encouraging perspiration to carry away waste products from the body. You can intensify the cleansing process by introducing stimulating essential oils, such as peppermint, pine, or geranium to the mix. You might like to sprinkle seaweed into a saltwater bath. It contains an amazing concentration of minerals and trace elements from the marine environment, and in baths of body temperature, the goodness of these constituents is thought to be taken up by the skin. Here also are recipes for exfoliating salt scrubs that leave skin silky smooth and with a soft glaze. Sea and Epsom salt baths are a recipe for a restful night's sleep. In the evening, relax in the water for 12 minutes, running the hot faucet as you lie there to speed perspiration. Sip a glass of mineral water to rehydrate. Climb out slowly and shower off any salt residue before retiring to bed in freshly laundered pajamas.

Caution: Avoid if you are pregnant, if you have heart disease, or if you have high blood pressure.

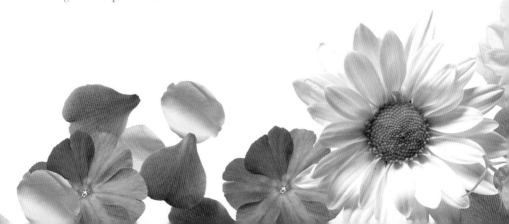

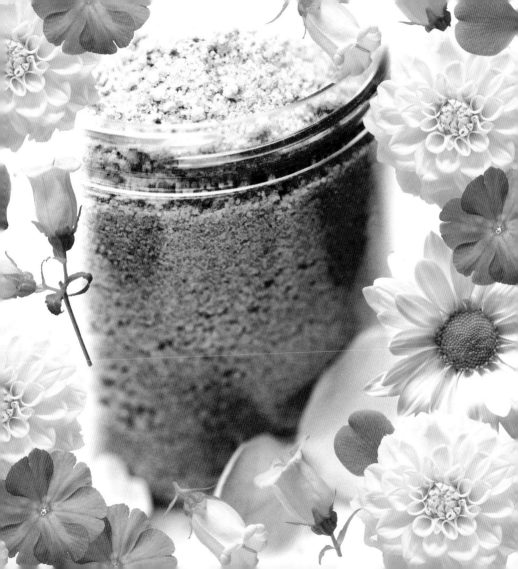

26   BASIC BATH SALTS

Ingredients

12 tbsp sea salt

Throw the salt into hot bathwater as the faucet runs. Additions might include
½ lemon or lime, freshly sliced, or up to ½ tsp food coloring or red beet juice.

27   PEP-UP SALTS

Ingredients

9 tbsp Epsom salts | 4 drops essential oil of peppermint
4 tbsp sea salt

Blend the salts in a large bowl and stir into a hot bath as it runs. Drop in the
peppermint oil just before stepping in, swishing to disperse.

28   CITRUS TONIC SALTS

Ingredients

12 tbsp Epsom salts | 2 drops each essential oils of
2 tbsp sunflower oil   grapefruit and basil

Blend the salts with the sunflower oil in a large bowl, then stir into a hot bath as
it runs. Drop in the essential oils just before stepping into the tub. Avoid sunlight
and sunlamps for 6 hours after use.

THAI BATH SALTS

Ingredients

6 tbsp sea salt | 3 drops each essential oils of
6 tbsp Epsom salts | lemongrass and ylang ylang

Mix the salts in a large bowl, then throw into a hot bath as the faucet runs. Drop in the essential oils just before stepping into the tub, swishing to disperse.

MEDITERRANEAN FOREST SALTS

Ingredients

12 tbsp sea salt | 3 drops each essential oils of pine
| and mandarin

Throw the salt into the bath as the hot water runs. Drop in the essential oils before stepping in, swishing to disperse. Avoid sunlight and sunlamps for 6 hours after use.

SEAWEED SALT SOAK

Ingredients

2 large strips dried kelp, dulse, | 12 tbsp seaweed-flecked sea salt
kombu, or nori seaweed | (look for Guérande *sel gris* or
6 tbsp dried mint | Breton *sel aux algues*)

Crumble the seaweed and place with the mint in a large pan of water. Bring to the boil, cover, and simmer for 30 minutes. Strain into a hot bath, then add the sea salt.

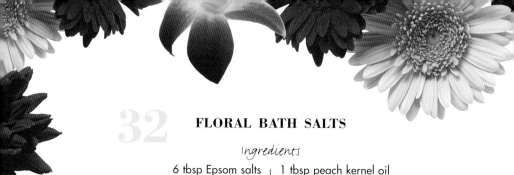

FLORAL BATH SALTS

Ingredients

6 tbsp Epsom salts	1 tbsp peach kernel oil
2 tbsp sea salt	3 drops each essential oils of rose,
4 tbsp baking soda	geranium, and lavender

Combine the salts and baking soda in a large bowl. Stir in the peach oil and throw into a hot bath as the faucet runs. Drop in the essential oils, swishing to disperse, just before stepping into the tub.

INDONESIAN SPICE SALTS

Ingredients

2 sticks cinnamon	6 drops essential oil of sandalwood
12 tbsp sea salt	1 drop essential oil of ginger

Break the cinnamon sticks and throw the pieces into a hot bath as you run the faucet. Then add the salt. Just before stepping into the tub, drop in the essential oils, swishing to disperse.

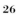

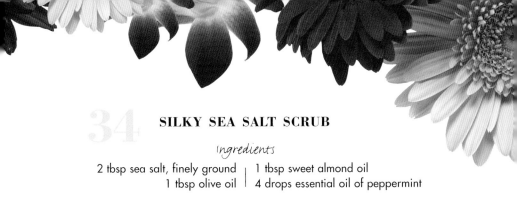

34 SILKY SEA SALT SCRUB

Ingredients

2 tbsp sea salt, finely ground | 1 tbsp sweet almond oil
1 tbsp olive oil | 4 drops essential oil of peppermint

In a large bowl, stir into the salt enough almond oil to make a medium-thick paste. Drop in the essential oil. Use as a body scrub, rubbing handfuls from heels to shoulders, or throw into a hot bath. Shower off. Omit peppermint oil if breast-feeding. If you have sensitive skin, do a patch test for peppermint oil before use.

35 SALT AND PEPPER BODY SCRUB

Ingredients

2 tbsp sea salt, finely ground | 2 tbsp honey
1 tsp freshly ground black pepper,
finely milled |

Mix together the salt and pepper in a large bowl, then stir in the honey. Massage handfuls over damp skin from heels to shoulders. Rinse off in a cool shower.

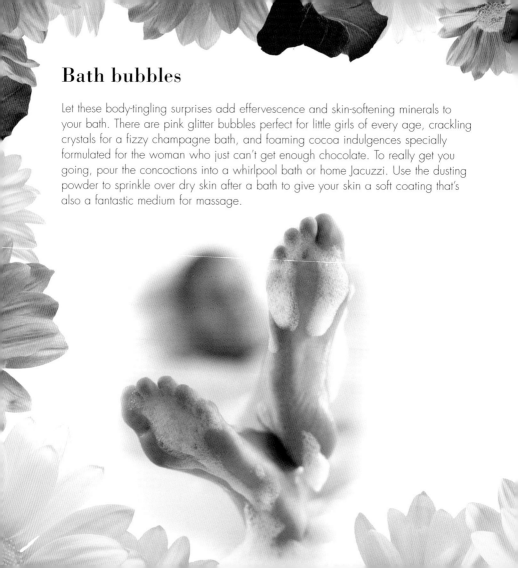

Bath bubbles

Let these body-tingling surprises add effervescence and skin-softening minerals to your bath. There are pink glitter bubbles perfect for little girls of every age, crackling crystals for a fizzy champagne bath, and foaming cocoa indulgences specially formulated for the woman who just can't get enough chocolate. To really get you going, pour the concoctions into a whirlpool bath or home Jacuzzi. Use the dusting powder to sprinkle over dry skin after a bath to give your skin a soft coating that's also a fantastic medium for massage.

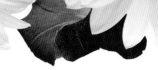

CHOCOLATE BUBBLE BATH

36

Ingredients

1 tbsp cocoa powder
2 tbsp heavy cream

1 tsp ground cinnamon
2 tbsp unscented shower gel

Mix the cocoa powder with enough of the cream to make a smooth thick paste. Stir in the cinnamon. Squirt the shower gel into a bowl and blend with the cocoa-cream mixture. Add to the bath as you run the faucet.

GLITTERY BATH BUBBLES

37

Ingredients

2 tbsp unscented shower gel
(for children, choose "green" products based on organic, nonsynthetic ingredients)

1 tbsp glitter body lotion
few drops pink food coloring or red beet juice

Stir together the shower gel and body lotion to create a glittery mix. Tint to the shade of pink you desire with the food coloring or beet juice. Add a good amount to a bath when turning on the faucet.

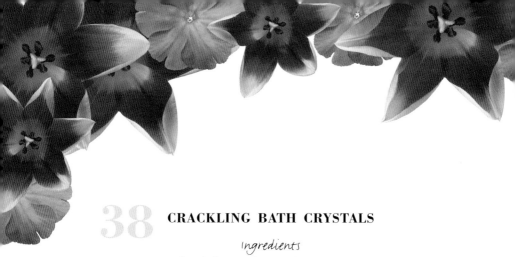

38   CRACKLING BATH CRYSTALS

Ingredients

6 tbsp baking soda
4 tbsp citric acid crystals
1 tbsp cornstarch

8 drops essential oil of frankincense
1 drop essential oil of ginger

Combine the baking soda, citric acid, and cornstarch in a large bowl, being careful to keep them dry. Scatter over the bathwater just before stepping in. Then drop in the essential oils, swishing to disperse. If you have sensitive skin, do a patch test for ginger oil.

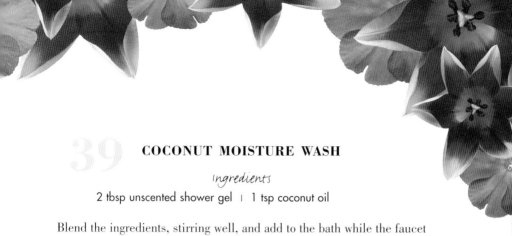

39   COCONUT MOISTURE WASH

Ingredients

2 tbsp unscented shower gel | 1 tsp coconut oil

Blend the ingredients, stirring well, and add to the bath while the faucet is running. Alternatively, use as a body wash in the shower.

40   VANILLA DUSTING POWDER

Ingredients

8 tbsp cornstarch | 4 drops vanilla essence

Place the cornstarch in a wide jar with a cover. Drop in the vanilla essence. Screw on the cover and shake to combine. Store in a cool dark place. To use, shake onto a powder puff and dust the skin, or pour into a flour shaker.

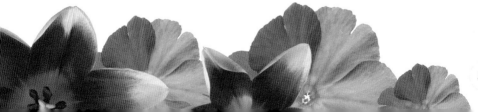

Bath buffs

Once a week before sinking into the bath, treat yourself to an exfoliating body scrub that lifts away impurities and polishes skin until it shines. We offer something for every skin type, from low-abrasion baby rice for sensitive souls to stimulating coffee for active men. The oil content in the scrubs leaves the skin with a super luster, even after showering, and essential oils contribute a lingering scent. After mixing the ingredients into a paste, massage handfuls into the skin, working up from heels to shoulders. For deeper exfoliation, briskly rub the area with a dampened loofah, if desired, making wide circular strokes in the direction of the heart. Relax for 10–20 minutes while the scrub dries like a mask, then rub off to remove the paste or take a refreshing shower. Don't forget to cover the drain with a strainer to collect the organic matter.

Caution: Avoid whole-body scrubs during pregnancy; steer clear of the products containing nuts if you have a nut allergy, cow milk products if you have a dairy allergy.

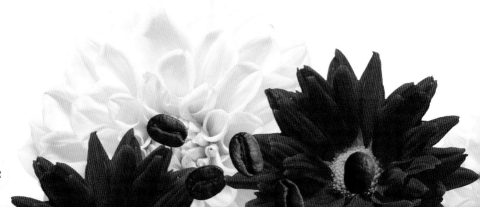

SESAME SEED POLISH

Ingredients

2 tbsp sesame seeds | 4 drops essential oil of peppermint
2 tbsp honey |

Stir the sesame seeds into the honey and drop in the essential oil. This mix makes a tingling moisture-rich foot scrub. Omit peppermint oil if breast-feeding; if you have sensitive skin, do a patch test for the oil.

MASCULINE COFFEE SCRUB

Ingredients

2 tbsp used coffee grounds (still warm) | 8 drops essential oil of frankincense
2 tsp granulated sugar | 2 drops essential oil of cardamom
2–3 tbsp olive oil |

Combine the coffee grounds and sugar. Stir in enough oil to produce a rather stiff paste. Drop in the essential oils. This mix is particularly good for back rubs, and men seem to find the aroma appealing. If you or the person you are massaging has sensitive skin, do a patch test for cardamom oil.

GENTLE RICE SCRUB

Ingredients

2 tbsp baby rice | 2 tbsp whole milk
1 tsp ground cinnamon | 6 drops essential oil of sandalwood
1 tsp ground almonds | 3 drops essential oil of patchouli

Mix the rice, ground cinnamon, and almonds. Stir in enough milk to make a smooth paste, adding the liquid little by little and stirring constantly to prevent lumps. Drop in the essential oils.

BOREH BODY RUB

Ingredients

2 tsp cloves | 1 tsp ground coriander
1 in (2.5 cm) fresh ginger root, finely grated | 1 tsp ground nutmeg
½ tsp ground cinnamon | 1 tbsp baby rice
| 3 tbsp sunflower oil

Pound the cloves and grated ginger using a pestle and mortar. Mix in the ground spices and rice, stirring well, then stir in enough of the oil to make a paste. Avoid if you have sensitive skin.

45 *LULUR* POWDER SCRUB

Ingredients

2 tbsp baby rice	6–8 tbsp whole milk
1 tsp ground turmeric	6 drops essential oil of jasmine
2 tsp ground ginger	2 drops essential oil of sandalwood

Combine the rice and spices, then moisten to a paste by adding the milk little by little, constantly stirring. Drop in the essential oils.

46 INDIAN BRIDAL *UBTAN* RUB

Ingredients

1 tsp cumin seeds	½ tsp grated nutmeg
1 tsp sesame seeds	1 tsp mustard oil
6 saffron strands	2 tbsp sesame seed oil
2 tbsp gram (garbanzo bean) flour	6 drops essential oil of sandalwood
½ tsp ground turmeric	4 drops essential oil of jasmine

Grind the cumin, sesame seeds, and saffron strands to a fine powder using a pestle and mortar. Stir in the gram flour, turmeric, and nutmeg, mixing well. Drizzle in the mustard oil and enough sesame oil to make a sloppy paste. Drop in the essential oils.

47 BALINESE COCONUT-TURMERIC SCRUB

Ingredients

1 coconut | 1 tsp turmeric powder

Crack open the coconut and grate the flesh. Stir in the turmeric
and rub handfuls into moistened skin.

48 FACIAL PESTO POLISH

Ingredients

2 large whole cashew nuts, unsalted | 1 drop each essential oils of geranium
1 tsp sesame seed oil | and vetivert
½ tbsp honey |

Pound the cashew nuts into a moist powder using a pestle and mortar. Mix in the
sesame oil little by little until combined, then stir in the honey vigorously. Drop
in the essential oils. Massage over face and neck, wipe away with a warm, wet
washcloth, then splash with tepid water, and tone. Omit geranium oil during
pregnancy; do a patch test if you have sensitive skin.

THAI POPPY SEED SCRUB

Ingredients

1 tbsp poppy seeds
2 tbsp honey
1 tbsp live natural yogurt

squeeze of fresh lemon juice
4 drops essential oil of lemongrass

Blend the poppy seeds and honey. Stir in the yogurt, then the lemon juice, to create a runny paste. If you have sensitive skin, do a patch test for lemongrass oil and lemon juice.

FLORAL FACE SCRUB

Ingredients

2 tsp fine oatmeal
2 tsp powdered milk
½ tsp sweet almond oil

1 tbsp rosewater
3 drops essential oil of rose
1 drop essential oil of geranium

Mix together the oatmeal and powdered milk, then stir in the almond oil. Blend to a paste using as much rosewater as desired. Drop in the essential oils. Massage into face and neck, wipe away with a warm, wet washcloth, then splash with cool water. Omit the essential oils during pregnancy. If you have sensitive skin, do a patch test for geranium oil.

Bath masks

Give up one evening a week before your bath to cover your body in mud, coat your face with chocolate or crushed grapes, sink your feet into honey, and slather your hair with mashed banana before plunging into a warm bath or sloughing away dead skin cells in the shower. Such face and body masks have been used across the world for centuries to purify the skin and moisturize. Clay draws impurities from the skin and replenishes it by imparting minerals and trace elements as it dries, while tropical fruits are packed with revitalizing vitamins and antioxidants that fight the free-radical damage that speeds signs of ageing. When showering after use, place a strainer over the drain.

Caution: Do not use full-body masks during pregnancy; avoid cow milk products if you are allergic to dairy.

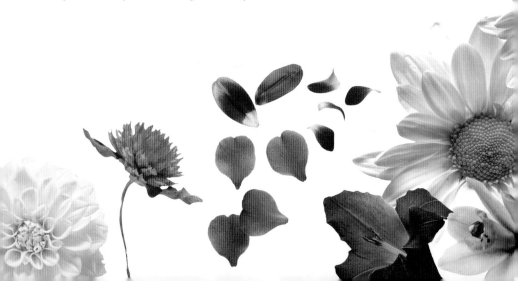

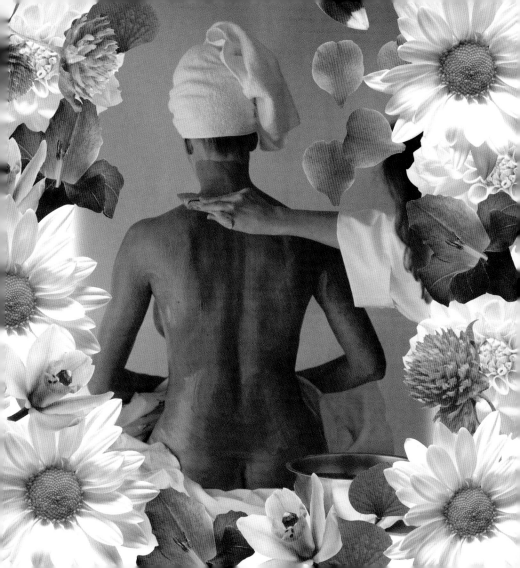

51   GRAPE FACIAL MASK

Ingredients

20 seedless red grapes | 1 tsp grapeseed oil
squeeze of fresh lemon juice | 1 egg white

Mix the grapes in a food processor until smooth, then add the lemon juice and the oil little by little. Whisk the egg white until frothy, then fold into the grape pulp. Apply to the face, avoiding the eye area, and relax for 15 minutes. Wipe away with a warm, wet washcloth, then splash with tepid water. If you have sensitive skin, omit the lemon juice.

52   CHOCOLATE FACE MASK

Ingredients

1 tsp honey | 1 tsp cocoa powder
1 tbsp heavy cream | 1 tsp fine oatmeal

Blend the honey and cream in a bowl, stirring continuously until they combine. Stir in the cocoa powder little by little until no lumps remain. Finally, mix in the oatmeal. Smear over the face, avoiding the eye area, and relax for 10 minutes. Wipe away the mask with a warm, wet washcloth, then splash the face with warm water.

HONEY FACIAL SILK

Ingredients

1 egg yolk	1 tsp sweet almond oil
2 tsp honey	1 vitamin E capsule

In a bowl, blend the egg yolk with the honey and oil, stirring constantly until combined. Prick the capsule and squeeze the contents into the egg mixture. Stir well. Apply to cleansed skin, avoiding the eye area. Relax for 15 minutes. Wipe away with a warm, wet washcloth, then splash with tepid water.

DETOX MOISTURIZING CLAY

Ingredients

1 ripe banana, peeled	3–4 tbsp Java or kaolin clay
1 ½ tbsp fine oatmeal	

Peel, mash the banana, and mix into the oatmeal in a large bowl. Stir in the dry clay, then add enough water to make a paste, adding the liquid little by little and mixing constantly to prevent lumps. Immediately rub handfuls onto face and neck, breast and underam area to make the most of its detoxifying and moisturizing properties. Allow to dry for 10–15 minutes, then remove with a warm, wet washcloth. Splash with cool water, then tone.

55 THAI HONEY BODY MASK

Ingredients

2 tbsp whole milk	2 in (5 cm) fresh ginger root, finely grated
4 tbsp thin honey	6 drops essential oil of jasmine

In a large bowl, stir the milk into the honey—be patient, it can take time to amalgamate. Once it has come together, mix in the grated ginger, then the jasmine oil. Dampen a natural sea sponge and dab the mask over the skin from heels to shoulders. Relax for 15 minutes, then wipe or shower off.

56 SPICED BODY CLAY

Ingredients

3 tbsp kaolin clay	2 drops each essential oils of fennel and
2 tsp sandalwood powder, if available	sandalwood
2 tsp cinnamon powder	

Mix the clay with the powdered spices in a large bowl. Pour in enough water to make a smooth paste, adding a little at a time and stirring constantly to prevent lumps. Drop in the essential oils. Smooth over the skin from heels to shoulders. Allow to dry for 20 minutes, then wipe or shower off. Omit fennel oil if epileptic and do a patch test for the essential oil if you have sensitive skin.

57   BANANA BODY MOISTURE MASK

Ingredients

2 very ripe bananas	4 tbsp thin honey
2 tbsp heavy cream	1 tbsp sea salt, finely ground

Peel and mash the bananas, then blend in the cream and honey, stirring well until amalgamated; use a food processor to save time. Stir in the salt and immediately rub into the skin, from heels to shoulders. Allow to dry for 20 minutes, then shower off.

58   COOLING CLAY MASK

Ingredients

4 tbsp Java clay, Dead Sea mud, or kaolin clay	3 drops each essential oils of jasmine, mandarin, and lavender
4-6 tbsp rose or orange blossom water	

In a large bowl, moisten the clay with the flower water until you achieve the consistency you prefer. Add a little of the liquid at a time, stirring constantly to prevent lumps. Drop in the essential oils, a blend renowned for softening stretch marks and scars. Smooth over the skin. Allow to dry for 20 minutes, then wipe or shower off. Avoid sunlight and sunlamps for 6 hours after use.

59 FOOT-SOFTENING MASK

Ingredients

1 tbsp thin honey | squeeze of fresh lemon juice
1 tbsp olive oil | 4 drops essential oil of black pepper

Mix the honey with the olive oil, stirring constantly until combined. Mix in the lemon juice and essential oil. Massage into feet, place each foot in a plastic bag, cover with a warm towel, and relax for 10 minutes. Wipe away the residue. If you have sensitive skin, do a patch test for the black pepper oil and lemon juice.

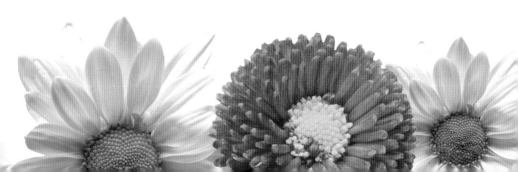

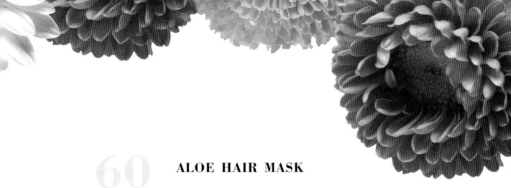

ALOE HAIR MASK

Ingredients

1 aloe vera leaf or 1 tbsp aloe gel
1 tbsp conditioner, according to
your hair type
4 drops essential oil of ylang ylang
for dry hair, 1 ripe peeled and mashed
banana and 1 tbsp coconut milk;

or for oily hair, 1 tbsp rosemary tea
(steep a tea bag in a cup of just-boiled
water for 10 minutes);
or for a flaky scalp, 2 tsp dried mint
and 1 tbsp thin honey

Score the aloe leaf and force out the gel with the back of a spoon, or squirt the gel from the tube. Stir into the conditioner, then add the essential oil. Mix in the extra ingredients according to your hair type. Massage into dry hair, manipulating the scalp as you work. Pile hair on your head, cover with a plastic shower cap, then wrap in a warmed towel for 20 minutes. Shower off, then wash and condition hair as usual.

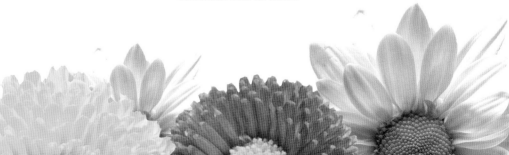

Bath bags and herbal potions

Petals look stunning floating on bathwater—just the sight of them can lift the spirits—but the detritus may clog your pipes. If you don't want to place a strainer over the drain as you empty the bath, make up muslin bath bags for herbs and flowers. For each bag you will need a piece of cheesecloth or muslin fabric approximately 9 in (23 cm) square. Pile the dried or fresh ingredients in the center and tie the corners together to secure. You can float the muslin bag beneath the faucet as you draw the bath, or suspend it with a little string beneath the hot faucet. Once the bath has run, use bags as an alternative to soap to wash your skin—much less drying than regular bath detergents. Here also are herbal infusions to strain into a bathtub or footbath before you sink in.

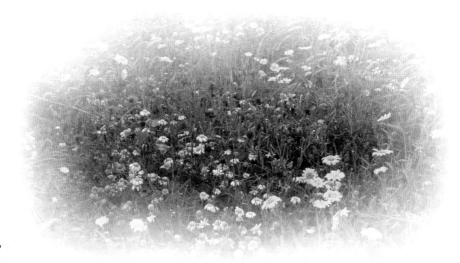

DEEP SLEEPING BAG

Ingredients

4 tbsp dried lavender flowers | 2 drops essential oil of clary sage
4 tbsp dried chamomile flowers |

Pile the herbs into the center of a square of muslin, drop on the essential oil, and
tie to secure. Suspend beneath the hot faucet while it runs or float it in the tub.
If drinking alcohol or driving omit clary sage oil.

OATMEAL SKIN SCRUB BAG

Ingredients

6 tbsp fine oatmeal | 6 tbsp dried rose petals, crushed

Pile the ingredients in the center of a square of muslin and tie to secure.
Float it in the tub while the faucet runs, then use in the bath to scrub the skin.

ZINGY ORANGE BATH BAG

Ingredients

grated zest of 1 orange | 2 in (5 cm) fresh ginger root, grated

Pile the ingredients in the center of a square of muslin and tie to secure.
Suspend beneath the hot faucet while it runs or float it in the tub.

MINTY FRESH BATH BAG

Ingredients

8 tbsp fresh (chopped) or 4 tbsp dried mint | 2 tbsp fresh rosemary needles
2 tbsp fresh or dried bay leaves

Pile the herbs in the center of a square of muslin and tie to secure. Throw into a bath when you run the water or suspend it beneath the hot faucet. Avoid if pregnant or breast-feeding.

SAFFRON INFUSION

Ingredients

10 strands of saffron

Place the saffron strands in a cup and pour just-boiled water over them. Allow to infuse for 20 minutes. Strain the saffron water into the bath just before stepping in.

GREEN TEA TONER

Ingredients

1 green tea bag | 2 drops essential oil of tea tree

Place the tea bag in a cup and pour just-boiled water over it. Allow to steep for 20 minutes, then remove the bag and drop in the essential oil. Soak a natural sea sponge or washcloth in the liquid, squeeze out, then use to tone skin after cleansing. Alternatively, use as a facial splash. If you have sensitive skin, do a patch test for tea tree oil.

67 FLOWER WATER SKIN SPLASH

Ingredients

3 tbsp rosewater
3 tbsp orange flower water
2 drops each essential oils of neroli,
petitgrain, lavender, and patchouli

1 drop each essential oils of rosemary,
orange, and clove

Combine the flower waters in a dark glass bottle. Drop in the essential oils, shake to combine, then use as a body splash (omit the essential oils during pregnancy) or decant into an atomizer for spraying towels or misting clothes while ironing.

68 MINT TONIC FOOT SOAK

Ingredients

2 tbsp dried mint

Place the mint in a cup and pour just-boiled water over it. Allow to steep for 20 minutes before straining into a footbath.

69 LIME HAIR TONIC

Ingredients

1 lime

Juice the lime and dilute in 1pt (600 ml) cool water. After shampooing, use the lime solution to rinse the hair; try to avoid the scalp if you plan to go outdoors or use a sunlamp for six hours (lime is a photosensitizing agent).

part two
Blissful baths

These are bathing treats to spoil you rotten and make your skin sparkle. Some of them offer inspiration for outdoor bathing expeditions—to the ocean, naturally heated spring water, or tropical pools. But most of the delights in store aim to replicate the rituals more and more of us choose to indulge in (or just aspire to) at beauty spas and health clubs around the globe, with signature spa treatments from Bali and Thailand, India and Japan. Each is more than a simple bath, featuring pampering body polishes or face masks, intensive oil treatments for the feet and nails, and repair care for the hair. Easy to follow, they use the home-spa products described in Part 1. Lock the door, turn off your phone, turn up the music, and enjoy a decadent evening indulging the person who deserves it most—that's you.

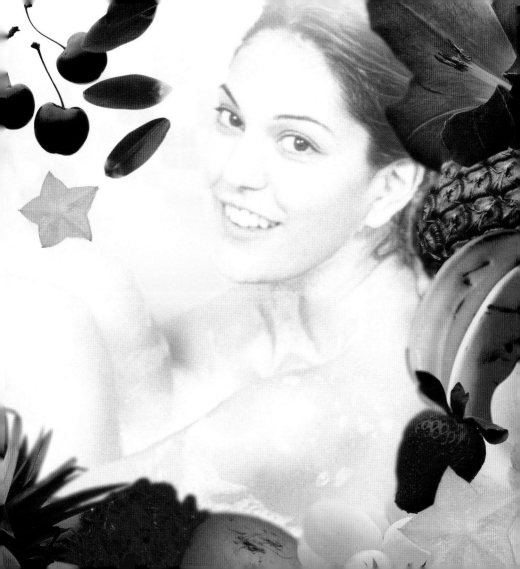

70 Bathing in flowers

What could feel more hedonistic than bathing in flowers? Use floral baths to keep you in touch with the seasons, like bathers in Japan, casting in cherry blossom in the spring, lavender and rose petals in midsummer, French marigolds in the fall. Or search for Japanese bath salts crafted artfully to echo the scents and colors of the seasons' flora. If gathering roses from your garden, pluck blooms just before sunrise when the life force within the dew-drenched plant is thought to be most potent. (By mid-morning, the essential oil content of rose petals plummets by 40 percent.) Or opt for exotic flowers from the florist, supplemented with a few drops of the matching essential oil. Heavy-scented jasmine, perhaps, which is especially softening in a bath for dry, sensitive skin. For me, this king of floral oils evokes south India, where in the early evening every street corner seems filled with baskets of jasmine strung into garlands to scent the hair. In Thailand, the flowers form part of Buddhist temple offerings and are exchanged as a symbol of friendship. In China, they stand simply for beauty. Or fly to the "New World" in a *florecida*, or flower bath, scented with vanilla, the dried seed pod of a Mexican orchid that flowers for just one day. These baths work beautifully outdoors in the sun; try a child's wading pool or a tin tub.

Caution: Omit bath milks if allergic to dairy products; during pregnancy avoid bath salts and jasmine and rose oils; if drinking alcohol or driving omit clary sage.

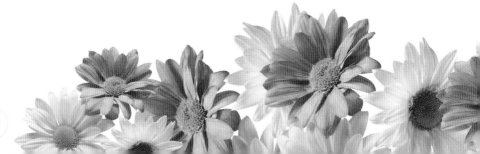

flower solution (see step 1 below)
or jasmine milk bath (page 17)
or floral bath salts (page 26)
or milk and rose petal bath bag
(page 19)

or deep sleeping bag (page 47)
or jasmine skincare oil (page 12)
oatmeal skin scrub bag (page 47)
flower water skin splash (page 49)
vanilla dusting powder (page 31)

1 If gathering roses to scent your bath, do so early in the day, while they are still covered in dew. Collect other flowers while the sun is at its height. Give thanks to the plant and to nature as you pluck it. Set blooms to soak in a wide glass bowl of water in sunlight for a few hours so they infuse the water with their scent and healing properties. Every 30 minutes, squeeze the plants to help them release their goodness.

2 Run a bath, throw in the soaked flower water, bath milk or salts, or one of the bath bags. Alternatively, pour in the bath oil just before stepping in.

3 Wash your skin with the oatmeal and rose scrub bag, rubbing gently to exfoliate with the milky secretions and muslin texture.

4 Step out of the bath. Shower off the salt residue if you took a salt bath. Pat dry with a soft fluffy towel, then splash your skin with the flower water and dust with the vanilla powder.

71   Bathing in scent

"Ointment and perfume rejoice the heart," states the Bible (*Proverbs 27: 9*). In warm water, the heart-gladdening effects of scent are more potent still. Heat makes aromas extra pungent—in a steamy bathroom, essential oils give off more aromatic molecules—and water-softened skin absorbs perfumed oils more rapidly. The perfumes used in this bath have been selected not just for their heavenly scent, but for their ability to bring joy and inner peace, sweeten a bad mood, and lift the spirits. They are all oils loved by perfumers. Ylang ylang, steam-distilled from the flowers of the tropical "perfume tree," has an exotic sweetness that encourages an almost euphoric joyfulness (aromatherapists say it relaxes the nervous system and regulates adrenaline flow). Spicy frankincense is a traditional aid to meditation, soothing the mind and lifting the spirits by deepening breathing. Richly floral jasmine is an energizing antidepressant, said to arouse feelings of positivity and self-confidence. Alternatively, try the milk bath inspired by ancient Egypt's famous fragrance *kyphi*, meaning "welcome to the gods." Like frankincense, which it included, this aroma is thought to draw the inhaler into a prayerful state (when burned, frankincense resin gives off a psychoactive substance). It also helps counter anxiety and insomnia while promoting a more cheerful state of mind. The components frankincense and myrrh are also fabulous skin conditioners. Enjoy this bath on dark evenings by candlelight; darkness seems to magnify the impressions of the scents.

Caution: Omit milk bath if allergic to dairy products; if pregnant omit jasmine, myrrh, and cypress oils; if you have sensitive skin, do a patch test for ylang ylang oil.

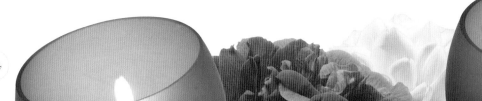

2 drops essential oil of jasmine
beeswax candles

joyful scent oil (page 12)
or Egyptian milk bath (page 21)

1 Press a freshly laundered robe and bath towel, scenting the water in the iron's reservoir with 2 drops essential oil of jasmine.

2 Light candles in the bathroom—beeswax has the best aroma.

3 Run a deep, warm bath. Add the bath oil or milk bath solution just before stepping in.

4 As you lie in the bath, close your eyes and test your sense of smell. Try to detect the individual notes within the scent. The first impressions you

detect are top notes. The body of the scent forms the middle notes, and the lingering character is referred to as base notes. Smoky myrrh and balsamic frankincense have lingering base notes, for example, while flowery ylang ylang shows strong top and middle notes. Try to discern too, the "tastes" sweet and sour, hot and bitter in the bath preparations.

5 Step out of the bath and pat dry. Don the scented robe and spend the rest of the evening drifting around the house wafting scent.

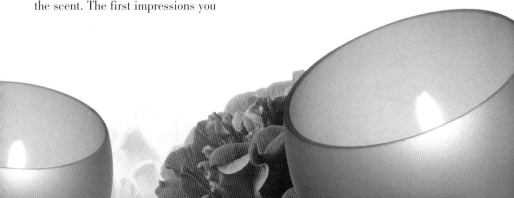

Bathing in color

Color therapists believe that bathing in colored water can restore harmony to a stressed body and mind. Certainly, color affects mood; research studies have shown that a yellow environment stimulates the ability to take in information, exposure to red light causes blood pressure and heart rates to rise, while blue light decreases them. Choose colors for your bath according to the effect you wish to achieve (see below). Different color baths work well at various times of the day: red, orange, and yellow invigorate in the morning; by evening you'll do better with more restful pastel tones of green, blue, indigo, and violet. Use a tiny amount of food coloring (up to ½ tsp) to tint your bath, or for more natural color substitute a little red beet juice.

• **Red** for physical energy, courage, sexual desire, stamina, potent revitalization, and inner strength. Avoid deep red when angry. Try pink to counter aggression. *Augment with 10 drops essential oil of rose.*

• **Orange** for creativity, positivity, and extreme invigoration. Counters inhibition and boosts confidence, productivity, and resourcefulness. Good before a challenging day at work. *Augment with 5 drops essential oil of orange. (Avoid sun and sunlamps for 6 hours after the bath.)*

• **Yellow** to stimulate the mind and relieve anxiety. Good for clarity of thought and a positive state of mind. *Augment with 3 drops essential oil of melissa. (If you have sensitive skin, do a patch test for this oil.)*

• **Green**, the universal color of healing and renewal; recommended for relaxation, concentration, inner peace, and reducing nervous and muscular tension. Good for promoting love. *Augment with 2 drops in total essential oil of cedarwood or pine. (If you have sensitive skin, do a patch test for these oils.)*

• **Blue** for soothing and mental relaxation. Good for treating fevers and colds and relieving insomnia. Use dark blue sparingly. *Augment with 5 drops in total essential oil of juniper. (Avoid if you have kidney disease.)*

• **Indigo** for soothing the nervous system, relieving insomnia, and boosting imagination. *Augment with 8 drops in total essential oil of frankincense or jasmine.*

• **Violet** for enhanced artistic creativity, perception, intuition, and head to toe rejuvenation. *Augment with 10 drops in total essential oil of geranium or lavender.*

Caution: Avoid if you have heart disease, high blood pressure, or are pregnant.

You will need:

basic bath salts (page 24) colored soap	Colored towels to match your bath, if desired

1 Fill a tall glass with mineral water. Wrap a sheet of colored gel (from photography shops) around it. Place in sunlight for an hour. Remove the gel.

2 Run a warm bath. Drop a few drops of food coloring into the basic salt solution. Start with a pastel shade, mixing in a little more color to deepen the hue. Beware of very dark colors; they can be overwhelming. Dissolve the colored salts in the bathwater.

3 Climb in and relax for 10 minutes. As you lie there, close your eyes and imagine breathing in the color as you inhale. Visualize it traveling to every part of the body that needs it. Sip the "colorized" mineral water when you need it. Wash with appropriately colored and scented soap.

4 Step out of the bath, shower off any salt residue, and wrap yourself in a towel of a corresponding color.

73   Bathing in wine

Drinking a daily glass of red wine is well known to be good for health, but bathing in the stuff? Soaking in extracts of grape skins—*Vinothérapie*—was invented, appropriately, in the Bordeaux region of France, and is said to help reduce wrinkles, nourish and lift sagging skin, and fight against cellulite. At the world's first wine spa in the fourteenth-century chateau les Sources de Caudalie, you can relax in a "Wine Barrel Bath"—a bubbling Jacuzzi of naturally hot spring water, its rich mix of minerals enriched with essential oils and the residue left over from grape pressing. Alternatively, be enveloped in a wrap made up from local honey, herbs, and wine; or sample a Sauvignon massage, crushed Cabernet body scrub, or Premier Grand Cru facial, all based on grapeseed residue. Research at France's University of Pharmacy in Bordeaux reveals grape extracts to have a high concentration of cell membrane-strengthening polyphenols. These compounds increase the strength of blood vessels by boosting microcirculation, protect elastin and collagen fibers, and prevent the destruction of the skin's support tissue. Grapeseed polyphenols are also 10,000 times more powerful than vitamin E at neutralizing skin-damaging free radicals. There are Caudalie day spas in Paris and Las Vegas, and spas specializing in wine therapy from Tuscany to Tasmania, California's Napa Valley to South Africa's Cape. Or base home treatments on grapeseed oil. Heat-extracted from the seeds of muscat grapes, it is particularly beneficial for oily skin. Of course, the must-have addition while you soak is a glass of Merlot, Cabernet, or Sauvignon. Cheers!

Caution: During pregnancy use only mandarin oil; if you have sensitive skin, do a patch test for pine and basil oils, and for lemon juice; avoid sunlight and sunlamps for 6 hours after bathing.

You will need:

grapeseed oil	grape facial mask (page 40)
your regular facial cleanser	wine bath oil (page 13)

1 Place the bottle of grapeseed oil in a pitcher of hot water to warm. Cleanse your face. Apply the grape mask, avoiding the eye area. Relax for 15 minutes, then wipe away with a warm, wet washcloth and splash the face with tepid water.

2 Run a warm, deep bath, pouring in the wine bath solution. Make sure the bathroom is well heated.

3 Before bathing, give yourself a grapeseed oil massage. Pour a little oil into the palm of one hand and rub your palms together. Make long sweeping strokes over your calves and thighs, arms and abdomen, shoulders and upper back.

4 Add more oil, if necessary, and knead fleshy areas, such as the thighs and buttocks. Use your thumbs to exert pressure into knotted muscles around your shoulders and neck. Adding more oil again if needed, finish with long soothing strokes down your arms, pulling away at the fingertips.

5 Step into the tub and relax for at least 20 minutes with a glass of your favorite wine and a French novel—try *Le Blé en Herbe* by Colette or *Madame Bovary* by Flaubert. Top off the hot water as the bath cools.

6 Climb out and pat your skin dry with a fluffy towel. Lie down and rehydrate with a tall glass of mineral water.

74   Bathing in milk

According to legend, Cleopatra loved to bathe daily in milk; the ladies of the palaces of central Java also swore by this beautifying formula. Milk baths are renowned not only for preparing the body for sensuous pleasure, but for soothing and softening sensitive skin, and imparting nutrients to sun- and stress-ravaged skin. Vitamin A in milk helps maintain healthy skin while the lactic acid in sour milk is an alphahydroxy acid, prized in the cosmetic industry for its exfoliating action, which is thought to make the skin look younger. The prebotic cultures in the yogurt face mask below exfoliate gently and amino acids impart moisture. Milk has long been associated with an ability to nourish the soul as it feeds the body; it is an auspicious holy substance in India, where it is regarded as a food fit for the gods, with an ability to promote calmness and meditation. This bath is a good way to start relaxing in the early evening, and makes a luxurious precursor to a night of passion.

Caution: Avoid if allergic to dairy products; during pregnancy omit jasmine and rose oils.

You will need:

facial milk cleanser of your choice
milk and rose petal bath bag
(page 19)
aphrodisiac milk bath (page 17)

small container live natural yogurt
floral-scented body milk of your choice

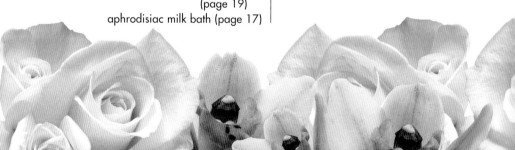

1 Draw a warm deep bath. Set a huge fluffy towel to warm on a radiator or heated towel rail. Cleanse your face using your regular cleansing milk.

2 Throw the milk and rose petal bath bag into the tub as the water runs. Then, just before stepping in, pour in the aphrodisiac milk bath solution. Swish well with your fingers to disperse.

3 Step into the tub and use the bath bag to cleanse your body. Massage your arms and legs, abdomen and back with the muslin, letting the milky secretions and scrubbing action exfoliate your skin and leave it smooth and silky.

4 Smear a layer of yogurt over your face and neck, avoiding the sensitive eye area. Relax for 15 minutes, topping off the hot water, if necessary, as the bath cools. Wipe away the face mask with a warm, wet washcloth, then splash with cool water.

5 When ready to climb out of the bath, wrap yourself in the warmed towel, and pat dry. While your skin is still a little damp, slather with copious amounts of body milk, then wrap yourself in a luxurious robe.

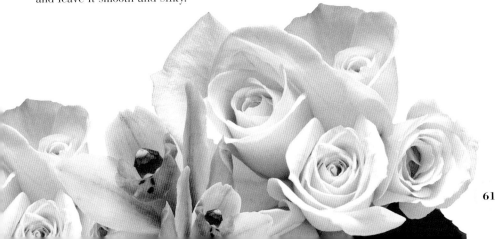

Bathing in honey

Another food of the gods, honey has a long history of use in beauty preparations to moisturize, nourish, and clarify the complexion while promoting suppleness and elasticity. Modern science is proving the efficacy of such folk beliefs, revealing the antimicrobial properties that make honey such a potent skin healer, able to soothe flare-ups at home and treat wounds, burns, or ulcers in hospitals. Honey rarely causes skin reactions, making it suitable for sensitive skins. The sticky nectar is rich in antioxidants that protect against cell damage caused by free radicals that contribute to signs of aging. The traditional Greek combination of yogurt and honey has more than taste going for it: honey has prebiotic properties, promoting in yogurt the growth of bifidobacteria (those valued in "prebiotic" products to support intestinal flora and suppress bad bacteria). A natural humectant, honey attracts moisture to the skin and seals it in, making it a recommended treatment for eczema in some hospitals. Levels of antioxidants and amino acids in honey vary according to the type of plant from which bees gathered nectar. Honey from bees fed herb extracts has been shown to have greater antioxidant activity, with honeydew honey from central European conifer forests and manuka honey from New Zealand having most antimicrobial action. Or select your honey for aroma and texture, and to reflect the flora of a region: lavender honey from Provence, France, orange blossom honey with its sweet, cloverlike aroma and beeswax texture, or sweet-scented but spicy Tupelo honey. Use once a week.

Caution: Avoid if allergic to dairy products; during pregnancy omit jasmine oil, lavender oil in the first trimester.

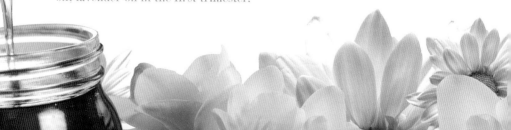

You will need:

milk and honey soak (page 19)
made with lavender honey
large sea sponge

Thai honey body mask (page 42)
your regular facial cleanser
honey facial silk (page 41)

1 Closing the bathroom door to retain warmth and moisturizing steam, run a deep, very warm bath, adding the milk and honey solution.

2 Moisten a large natural sea sponge. Dip it in the Thai mask and apply all over the body, focusing on areas that need extra moisture, such as the heels, knees, and elbows. Relax for 15 minutes, lying on an old towel.

3 Remove your makeup and cleanse your face following your regular cleansing routine.

4 Without wiping away the body mask, step into the bath and enjoy the heat and milky texture. Stroke your skin to loosen the mask. For an extra treat, snack on a bowl of Greek yogurt with a good spoonful of honey and some toasted sunflower seeds. Your insides will be as beautiful as your outside!

5 Apply the silky honey face mask, avoiding the delicate eye area. Relax for 15 minutes. Wipe away with a warm, wet washcloth, then splash with tepid water. Step out of the bath and pat dry.

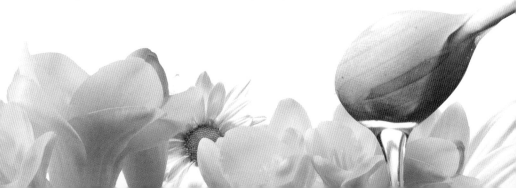

Bathing in chocolate

Forget the old wives' tales about chocolate giving you pimples; cocoa is the new must-have beauty ingredient. It is rich in flavonols, very potent antioxidant nutrients that help zap molecules known as free radicals associated with the aging process. It's also a great source of iron, copper, and magnesium to keep blood cells well oxygenated and muscles and nerves functioning. "Frrrozen Hot Chocolate" bath potions, the signature bodycare product of Serendipity restaurant in New York—long-renowned haunt of chocoholics including Marilyn Monroe and Grace Kelly—are flying out of stores. If you can't get to this chocolate Mecca, or to the other haunt of chocolate fiends in the United States, the Hershey spa, console yourself by wallowing in a chocolate bath at home. To maximize the benefits, nibble chilled chocolate truffles in summer, and sip a heartwarming hot chocolate drink in winter. Look, too, for chocolate-scented soup or melting bath bon bon bombs, or add the chocolate bubble bath recipe on page 29 to a whirlpool bath and climb in for a frothy moccacino. Laura Esquivel's novel *Like Water for Chocolate* makes the perfect accompaniment.

Caution: Avoid if you are allergic to dairy products; if you have sensitive skin, do a patch test for peppermint oil and omit if pregnant or breastfeeding.

You will need:

chocolate vanilla milk bath (page 18)	your regular facial moisturizer
your regular facial cleanser	peppermint foot cream (page 15)
orange flower water	vanilla dusting powder (page 31)
chocolate face mask (page 40)	

1 Run a very warm full bath. As the tub fills, mix up the chocolate vanilla milk and pour under the faucet.

2 Cleanse your face well, then tone by soaking a washcloth in hot water containing a little orange flower water. Squeeze, then sweep over your face. Pat dry.

3 Apply the creamy face mask, smoothing it over your cheeks, forehead, and chin, avoiding the delicate skin around the eyes. Resist the temptation to eat the mask!

4 Check the temperature and sink into the cocoa-scented water. Eat a truffle or two as you start to relax—choose those with a high proportion of cocoa solids—72 percent is the most delicious and healthful.

5 After 10 minutes, wipe away the mask with a warm wet washcloth, then tone again by soaking a washcloth in orange flower water as before.

6 Relax a little longer in the bath, if desired. When ready step out of the bath and pat dry. Moisturize your face, then anoint your feet with the peppermint cream (you might like to pop an edible peppermint cream into your mouth at this point).

7 To complete the good-enough-to-eat combination, dust skin with the vanilla scented powder, preferably using a supersized powder puff.

77 Bathing outdoors

Rotenburo, a Japanese outdoor bath in naturally heated spring water, translates literally as "a bath amid the dew under an open sky." All my best bathing experiences have been outdoors: aged seven in a muddy creak with jam sandwiches; in the "devil's cauldron" beneath a waterfall fed by icy mountain streams in Spain; in a rainforest in Java, swinging on Tarzan vines into a hidden pool; in a wintry Norwegian forest, the water a primeval inky black; in a steamy pool overlooking the Baltic Sea, body in warm water, head in icy air; in Pamukkale, Turkey, sitting in a shallow basin of spring water on the edge of a clifftop resembling frozen cascades of dazzling white cotton wool; in the crashing surf of the North Cornish coast; in my own garden with my daughters in an old tin tub. Wherever you are, get out there and take to the waters, braving the icy winds and whatever the seasons throw at you for one of the best sensations there could be—the feel of rock and mud underfoot, the crash of water tumbling, and the thrill of the wild!

Great outdoor bathing spots

- **Rauhaniemi sauna, in Tampere, Finland:** A popular public sauna where you can bathe from a hole in a frozen lake in the dark of winter.

- **The beaches of the Vänern archipelago near the city of Karlstad in Sweden:** Lake Vänern is Europe's largest freshwater lake; one can even bathe in the center of the city.

- **Blue Lagoon geothermal outdoor spa, in Iceland:** Sitting in milky blue, very hot mineral-rich water in a snowstorm is quite something.

- **Idaho Springs, Colorado:** Find the geothermal cave baths at the Indian Springs Resort first used by Ute and Arapahoe Indians.

- **Japanese outdoor *onsen* spa resorts:** Hoshi and Takaragawa in the mountains of Gunma Prefecture or Myogaya in the Kanomata River gorge in Tochigi Prefecture are considered among the most spectacular.

- **Thermal baths, Vals, Graubünden, Switzerland:** Amazing modern architecture hewn from local quartzite and concrete in a remote Alpine village housing thermal baths.

- **Budapest, Hungary:** The city has the highest number of medical thermal springs in one place in the world—more than 100 natural springs and 24 baths.

- **Aphrodite's Rock on the beach at Pafos, Cyprus:** Where the Greek goddess of love is said to have risen from the surf. Visit also the nearby dramatic Baths of Aphrodite, where the ancient world bathed outdoors, and the Fontana Amorosa.

- **The Source Spa in Bali:** Water gardens overlooking the holy Ayung River, where you can float in pools of pure mountain spring water to which pilgrims have always come for spiritual sustenance.

Safe outdoor bathing

If you're worried about the risks of bathing outdoors, look for beaches certified clean. These should have been tested for bacterial contamination, chemicals and other materials in the water, be far from sewage outlets, and have toilet facilities, trash cans, and life-saving facilities including a first aid kit and emergency telephone. Be aware of tide times, look for flags designating safe areas to swim, and ask locals about dangerous currents and tides. Don't swim in open water unless you are a strong swimmer, and don't dive in. If you are bathing alone, tell someone where you are going and when you should be back. Always enter the water via a slope or bank to ensure you can get out again.

78 Bracing sea bathing

Around the world on special days such as Christmas and New Year's, people from Cornwall in the UK to Australia run into the sea for good luck, good health, and the sheer intoxication of splashing in ocean waves! Dashing into an icy-feeling sea when you are warm boosts endorphins—natural opiates—and the greater the variance in temperature, the more stimulating and euphoric the effect. So healthy was ocean water considered in eighteenth- and nineteenth-century Europe that sea-bathing institutions were built to treat diseases like tuberculosis, asthma, and depression. From England, the sea bathing craze spread to French resorts with their outdoor "rolling bathtubs" or bathing huts. Modern French sea bathing establishments claim that it is impossible to mimic the beneficial qualities of seawater at home. However much salt and seaweed you add to a bath, you miss out on traces of phytoplankton thought to have an antibacterial action on skin. Six days of seaside cure twice a year are recommended by French thalassotherapy centers as the optimum time for refreshment and rejuvenation. So for ultimate well-being, head to the coast for a dip in the ocean and try out this stimulating exercise routine. Then take a long walk to breathe in the electronegative ions said to be charged with beneficial trace elements that effectively destress the body.

You will need:

lots of huge fluffy towels | vacuum flask filled with a warming drink, such as creamy hot chocolate

1 Run into the sea. Plunge your wrists and hands in, splash water over your shoulders, and immerse yourself. If it's cold keep swimming, or jumping up and down until you feel warmer.

2 Standing waist high in the water, boost your heart rate by doing star jumps: bend your knees until your shoulders are beneath the water and jump with your feet to the side and together, taking your arms to the water surface and down to your sides again. Follow with "spotty dogs," jumping feet forward and back and pushing alternate arms forward and back.

3 Bring your knees together. Jump with your feet and knees in one direction and take your arms and head to the other side. Alternate, jumping right and left.

4 Jog, bringing your knees up high, then taking heels to buttocks. Jumping, raise one knee, lifting it through the water to meet the opposite elbow. Alternate sides again.

5 Bend your knees to lower yourself in the water. With flexed hands, palms facing forward, push the water away, then pull it back toward you with cupped palms. Repeat the movements.

6 Bend your elbows, tucking them into your waist. With rounded palms, pull water toward your shoulders in a tricep curl. Then, turn your palms to face backward and take your forearms

behind you in a bicep extension. With arms outstretched, palms rounded, scoop your palms toward each other in front of your chest, turn your wrists and scoop out again, and repeat, as if doing breaststroke.

7 Stand with one foot behind the other and press through the back heel to stretch the calf. Hold. Stretch your quadricep by holding heel to buttock. Repeat on the other leg.

8 Interlinking fingers, press your palms forward and hold, feeling the stretch in your shoulder blades. Press your palms toward the sky, and hold. Bend one elbow and press it back with your other hand, trying to take the lower palm between your shoulder blades. Repeat on the other arm. Interlink fingers behind your back and stretch your arms toward the sky. Hold. Take one arm across your chest, pressing the upper arm with your free hand. Hold. Repeat on the other arm.

9 Wade out and briskly rub dry. Wrap up well and have a warming drink.

79 Midsummer mint cooler

A restorative footbath for aching, perspiring feet, this bathing treat is especially welcome in summer, when dirty sandal-clad feet really benefit from the good scrub the exfoliant provides. Peppermint is especially good for hot, itchy feet because of its antibacterial and antifungal actions, and its ingredient menthol, which has a cooling, anesthetizing effect on skin. The herb has long been used as a nerve tonic, to revive, refresh, and stimulate the senses; the Roman writer Pliny the Elder recommended wearing a crown of mint leaves to boost concentration. Use this footbath treatment as a wake-up call for the brain when you have to get up and go on sultry summer afternoons; sipping a cup of peppermint tea as you wallow in the footbath can make you feel instantly more alert. This bathing treatment includes a moisturizing and softening honey and olive oil foot mask plus an easy yoga exercise to banish swelling around the feet and ankles and guard against varicose veins. This very restorative pose also relieves exhaustion by boosting circulation to the upper body. This is a great calming and rejuvenating bath treatment.

Caution: Avoid peppermint while pregnant or breast-feeding; if you have sensitive skin, do a patch test for black pepper and peppermint oils, and for lemon juice.

You will need:

peppermint tea bag
mint tonic foot soak (page 49)
sesame seed polish (page 33)

pumice stone
foot softening mask (page 44)

1 Place the tea bag in a cup and pour just-boiled water over it. Steep for 5 minutes. Fill a bucket with tepid water. Strain in the mint tonic foot soak, then sit on a chair with the bucket in front of you and plunge in both legs up to the knee. Relax for 15 minutes, sipping the peppermint tea. Pat dry with a fluffy towel.

2 To reduce swelling and boost *joie de vivre*, try this yoga semi-inverted posture. Lie on your back with your buttocks against a wall, legs up against the wall, knees slightly bent. Shuffle yourself in until both buttocks firmly touch the wall. Relax your arms to the side, palms open and facing upward. Try to straighten your calves with each out-breath, pressing through the heels and edges of the feet, as if supporting a weight, and feeling the stretch in the back of the calf. Hold for 3 minutes or more, relaxing the back of the neck and small of the back toward the ground. To exit the pose, bend your knees toward your chest and roll onto one side.

3 Get up slowly. Take handfuls of the sesame seed polish and scrub your feet, using more abrasive actions where you find hard skin. Plunge your feet back in the footbath to rinse away the sesame seeds. Dry your feet. Use a pumice stone around the heel and ball of the foot to remove stubborn dry skin, if necessary.

4 Apply the foot-softening mask, massaging it well into the heels, balls, between the toes, and into the nails. Place a plastic bag over each foot and wrap the feet in a warm towel. Relax for another 10 minutes. Have another cup of tea, if desired. Wipe away the residue with the towel and wiggle your tingling fresh honey-softened toes.

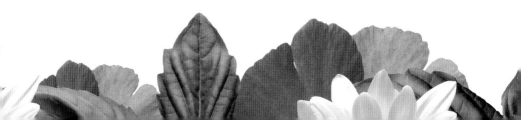

80 Footbath and pampering pedicure

When's the best time to give yourself a pedicure? When your feet have been softened and scented in a footbath, of course. Try this citrus-flavored milky foot soak to soften hard skin. Then polish away dry skin with a Thai-inspired exfoliator. Both products contain lemongrass; this acts not just as a whole-body reinvigorating tonic with its sharp citrus scent, but can ease away aches and tiredness, and deal with sweaty feet and fungal problems. It also helps reduce the fluid retention that may cause swollen ankles. The lemon and ginger moisturizer is warming for the extremities—ginger and lemon are both good circulation boosters—with ginger helping combat strained feet and refreshing lemon to soften brittle nails. Remove old nail polish before you start, looking for products marked as acetone-, toluene-, or formaldehyde-free for peace of mind; many nail polish removers contain these petrochemicals, some of which have been linked with cancer. Use once a week.

Caution: Omit milk powder if you are allergic to dairy products; omit geranium oil during pregnancy; if you have sensitive skin, do a patch test for lemon, ginger, and lemongrass oils, and lemon juice.

You will need:

nail polish remover
nail file, nail brush, orange stick,
pumice stone, chamois
lemongrass milk bath bag (page 21)
wide flat pebbles, optional

Thai poppy seed scrub (page 37)
2 pomegranates
lemon and ginger foot massage oil
(page 15)

1 Remove old nail polish. Soak a cotton ball in nail polish remover and sweep it from cuticle to tip.

2 File nails with a nail file, making long strokes in one direction only, working in from the outer edges. Keep the tips flat.

3 Sit back, relax, and plunge your feet into a bucket of warm water containing the bath bag. For an optional treat, heat some wide flat pebbles in a low oven until very warm, then place in the bucket beneath your feet. Read a book or listen to some music for 10 minutes. Sip an herbal tea. If your toenails are dirty, scrub with a nail brush. Pat dry.

4 Wrap a cotton ball around an orange stick and carefully push the cuticles back from each nail.

5 Massage in the Thai scrub. Rub well around the heels and balls of the feet, common areas of dryness.

6 Rinse your feet in the footbath. Pat dry, paying attention to the often-neglected area between the toes. Use a pumice stone to remove remaining dry skin, if necessary, sweeping in one direction only.

7 Halve each pomegranate and scoop out the seeds. Rub the seed-laden flesh over the feet, then place each foot in a plastic bag and wrap in a warm towel. Raise your feet and relax for another 10 minutes.

8 Rinse feet again in the footbath and dry well. Buff nails with a chamois, then moisturize your feet with the ginger foot oil, not neglecting the skin between each toe. Finally, rub a little oil into each nail, squeezing each one so nourishing oil slips into the gap between nail and cuticle.

9 Wait 15 minutes for the oil to absorb, then slip on cashmere socks or your favorite sexy sandals.

81 Nail bath and natural manicure

Neighborhood nail salons with their rush and bustle, acrylic extensions, and overpowering fumes are hardly relaxing places. This home manicure is an all-natural affair and makes your home a haven of peace. It uses only gentle ingredients (milk, clay, oil) to cleanse, scrub, and moisturize hands and nails—the part of the body most exposed to the elements and one that really benefits from a little time and attention. The treatment features a spicy hand mask to bring nutrients to chapped hands and worn, brittle nails. This is followed by an intensely moisturizing massage with an oil balm that's particularly emollient for dry hands; it contains sandalwood to work on dehydrated skin and damaged nails, and patchouli to help heal dry, cracked skin. Remove old nail polish before you start, looking for products free of acetone (linked with irritation to the nose, throat, lungs, and eyes). Try also to avoid formaldehyde, banned in Sweden and Japan, and toluene—the U.S. Protection Agency's Office of Pollution and Prevention Toxins warns that breathing it in quantities can affect the kidneys, liver, and heart. Use once a week.

Caution: Omit jasmine and fennel oils during pregnancy, lavender during the first trimester, fennel if epileptic; if you have sensitive skin, do a patch test for fennel oil; omit powdered milk if you are allergic to dairy products.

You will need:

nail polish remover	spiced body clay (page 42), make
nail file, nail brush, chamois,	up half the quantity
orange stick,	Eastern moisture balm (page 13)
milk and honey soak (page 19),	
make up half the quantity	

1 Remove old nail polish. Soak a cotton ball in nail polish remover and sweep from cuticle to tip.

2 File nails with a nail file, making long strokes in one direction and working inward from the outer edges. For a natural look, shape nails into a rounded oval, or straighten the tip to a blunt edge to strengthen nails.

3 Sit back and relax for 5 minutes as you soften hands and nails in a basin of warm water containing the milk and honey soak. Pat dry.

4 Wrap a cotton ball around an orange stick and carefully clean away dirt from beneath each nail. Wrap another cotton ball around the orange stick and gently push the cuticles back.

5 Cover your hands in the spicy clay, then place each one in a plastic bag and wrap in a warm towel. Lie down for 10 minutes.

6 Rinse your hands in the nail bath and pat dry. Buff nails to a high shine with the chamois, then pour a little of the moisture balm into one palm and warm between both palms. Interlink your fingers, rubbing palms together.

7 Supporting the palm of one hand with the fingers of the other hand, circle the middle of the palm with your thumb, warming the energy center here. Make the circle wider to cover the entire palm. Turn the hand over, add a little more oil, and, still supporting with your fingers, slide your thumb from the base of the fingers toward the wrist, working along each channel. Repeat.

8 Massage the thumb and fingers from base to tip, using your other thumb and index finger like a corkscrew. Squeeze at the tip as you pull your fingers away.

9 Repeat steps 7–8 on the other hand. Interlink your fingers again, rubbing the webs, then palms together. Finally, rub a little oil into each nail, squeezing each one so a little of the oil slips into the gap between nail and cuticle.

82   Hair repair cream bath

Try this once a week repair treatment for dull, lackluster locks on bad hair days.
It includes an energizing scalp massage to release tension and boost circulation—
Japanese hairdressing schools teach that washing and massage are as important
as a good cut in revitalizing the look of hair—and a hair mask popular in Asia for
strengthening hair shafts and revitalizing the scalp. The coconut conditioning oil
used for the massage contains fatty acids that resemble those of skin sebum and is
particularly good for dry hair and scalps. Add a ripe banana to the hair mask and
you have the benefits of tryptophan, a skin- and hair-strengthening amino acid. The
mask is fragranced with ylang ylang, a traditional scalp tonic thought to rebalance
sebum on dry and oily scalps alike. It is used in hair preparations around the world
to stimulate hair growth, as is aloe vera, which Indian women swear is the best
treatment for dark shiny tresses.

Caution: Omit lavender oil during the first trimester of pregnancy; if you
have sensitive skin, do a patch test for ylang ylang oil.

You will need:

coconut hair-conditioning oil (page 14)	aloe hair mask (page 45)
bath bag of your choice (pages 19, 21, 46–49)	shampoo and conditioner for your hair type
	sandalwood incense

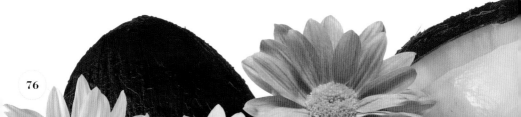

1 Start with dry hair. Warm the hair conditioning oil by standing the bottle in a bowl of hot water for a few minutes. Pour a little into the palm of one hand, then rub your hands together.

2 Place your fingertips at your hairline, little fingers touching at the center. Keeping your fingers stiff, knuckles bent, make small circles that move the tissue beneath the surface of the skin. Repeat 3 or 4 times, moving back an inch each time.

3 Apply more oil. Place your hands at the back of your head, fingers curled, little fingers at your temples, thumbs at the nape of your neck. Repeat the circling action, working your thumbs into knotted muscles at the neck. Move up the head an inch and repeat. Move up and repeat 3 or 4 times.

4 Apply more oil. Starting at the crown of the head, grasp handfuls of hair at the roots. Swiftly tug, hold, twist around your fingers, then pull away, shaking your hands. Repeat,

moving down the sides of the head. Repeat, starting at the hairline above your eyes and moving up and over the back of the head. This is thought to increase circulation to hair follicles.

5 To finish, comb your fingers through the hair on either side of the head, working from front to back.

6 Run a warm bath, suspending the bath bag beneath the hot faucet. Work the hair mask into your hair from the roots down, massaging the formula through to the very ends. Pile the messy hair on your head, cover with a shower cap, and wrap in a warm towel.

7 Relax in the scented bath for 20 minutes as the hair mask takes effect. Shower off the hair mask, keeping the water tepid to avoid "cooking" the brew. Wash and condition hair as usual, finishing with a cool-water rinse.

8 When hair is almost dry, carefully tousle it over the smoke from the incense stick to impart a lovely scent.

83   Relaxing bath time facial

This 20-minute treatment for tired skin carried out while you recline in a bath includes incredibly gentle massage known as manual lymph drainage that encourages the body's natural waste-disposal system, removing toxins and permitting optimum transmission of nutrients to cells. The technique helps alleviate puffy skin, and is also effective for under-eye bags. The smooth slow movements created in the 1930s by the Danish founders of this therapy, Dr. Emil Vodder and wife Estrid, are incredibly soporific. Vetivert is known as the oil of tranquillity because of its mind-calming and stress-relieving properties. The orange and ginger in the bath bag augment the detoxification, encouraging perspiration to carry away waste products from the body while boosting circulation. Their reviving scents will promote get-up-and-go: essential oil of orange lifts and revives, bringing about a new sense of energy and positivity; sharp spicy ginger augments this cheerful zest for life. Use once a week.

Caution: Avoid the pesto polish if you are allergic to nuts; omit rose oil during pregnancy, chamomile in the first trimester.

You will need:

zingy orange bath bag (page 47)	sea sponge
chamomile tea bag	facial pesto polish (page 36)
skin-cleansing oil (page 14)	your regular daytime facial moisturizer

1 Run a warm bath, throwing in the orange bath bag. Place the teabag in a cup and pour in boiling water. Leave to steep for 20 minutes. Meanwhile, apply a little of the skin-cleansing oil to a cotton ball. Wipe over the face, repeating until your face feels clean.

2 Soak a natural sea sponge in the chamomile tea, squeeze, and wipe over the face, cleansing away traces of oil. Then, scrub the entire face and neck with the pesto polish, making small circles with your fingertips.

3 Soak the sea sponge again in the chamomile tea, squeeze out, and wipe away the scrub. Before climbing into the bath, throw in the remaining skin-cleansing oil and swish to disperse.

4 In the bath, begin the slow massage strokes. Lying with your head resting on a small folded towel, raise your elbows out of the water and place your palms at the top of your neck, one on each side, fingers straight. Very slowly, manipulating skin only, not the muscle beneath, move your arms to smooth your palms up and back to form the start of a circle. Ease the pressure as the skin returns to its position naturally. Repeat four times.

5 Cross your arms and place palms on opposite shoulders. Repeat the gentle circle, moving the skin upward and out, and letting it come back to position naturally. Repeat 4 times.

6 Place your palms on each side of your jaw. Make 5 slow gentle circles, moving your arms to take the skin down and toward the ears, and letting it come back to position by itself. Move slightly toward the ears and repeat. Move again and repeat 3 times.

7 Place flattened relaxed fingers with the tips on either side of your mouth. Make 5 static circles as before. Move your fingers up, so the tips sit on your cheekbones. Make 5 circles in the same inert way, but with much less pressure. Move slightly toward the ear and repeat. Move and repeat again.

8 Place straight fingers gently over your forehead, tips in the center. Make 5 gentle circles, being careful to make the movements completely superficial. Move outward slightly and repeat. Move outward again, forefingers on temples, and repeat.

9 Step out of the bath completely relaxed and uplifted, and gently pat yourself dry. Apply your regular daytime moisturizer.

Green tea facial bath

This facial treatment offers complete regeneration. Green tea is one of nature's most potent health tonics, and has been seized upon by skincare gurus for its age-defying qualities. The skin-protective secrets of green tea derive from its high levels of antioxidants. These block the activity of free radicals that are implicated in disease and aging, and are potentially cancer-causing. This facial bath is also a great wind-down skin treat. If you prefer, substitute the tea bags over the eyes with off-the-shelf eye-contour patches formulated to reduce dark circles and tighten puffy skin.

Caution: Avoid sunlight and sunlamps for 6 hours after using the clay. Omit jasmine, rose, and geranium oils during pregnancy, lavender in the first trimester.

You will need:

2 green tea bags
sea sponge
1 tbsp rosewater
your regular facial cleanser
floral face scrub (page 37)
green tea toner (page 48, omit the
tea tree oil if you have sensitive skin)

facial massage blend for your
skin type (page 14)
cooling clay mask, mixed with warm
green tea instead of flower water
(page 43), make up half the quantity
gel-filled eye mask, chilled
your regular facial moisturizer
2 drops essential oil of rose

1 Place each tea bag in a cup of just-boiled water. Steep for 10 minutes. Run a bath, pouring in the green tea. Squeeze the tea bags and reserve. Soak a sea sponge in hot water scented with the rosewater. Cover your face in cleanser, using your fingertips to massage it over every part, starting to warm your skin. Squeeze out the sponge and wipe away the cleanser.

2 Massage your face and neck with the oatmeal scrub, working with tiny up and down movements into the sides of the nose, over the chin, and between the eyebrows—common sites for pimples and blackheads. Wipe away with the rosewater-soaked sponge. Then tone your face by splashing with the green tea toner.

3 Warm a little of the facial massage blend between your palms. Rest your hands over your face, without pressing on your eyes. Gently pull out from the center of your face to your hairline. Repeat. Sandwich your chin between your index fingers and thumbs. Draw out and up the jawline three times.

4 Apply a little more oil. Rest your fingertips on the side of your nose, then draw out over the cheekbones to circle the eye sockets. Continue toward the center of the eyebrows and glide down the bridge of the nose. Repeat the circling motion a few times.

5 Rest the tips of your middle fingers on the point at which your eyebrows begin, above the inner corner of each eye. Gently "saw" up and down, then stroke one finger in a diagonal line toward the top of your hairline. Repeat with the other finger, alternating strokes to build up a smooth repetitive crisscross over your forehead.

6 Rest fingertips in the center of your brow and pull outward. Repeat. Finally, massage your earlobes.

7 Apply the clay mask to your face and neck, avoiding the eyes and mouth. Lie back, placing the cooled tea bags over your eyes. Rest a gel-filled eye mask over them. Relax for 15 minutes.

8 Remove the tea bags and discard. Wipe away the mask with the soaked sponge again. Soak a clean washcloth in very hot water containing 2 drops essential oil of rose. Wring out, check that the temperature is not too hot, then place over your face. When it cools, wipe over the face and remove. Step out of the bath, pat dry, and apply your regular facial moisturizer.

85   Sun-repair clay treatment

Glorious mud—nothing quite like it for cooling the blood, goes the song. When you've spent too long in the sun, chill and restore your skin with this clay bathing treat. Eastern spas may recommend kaolin-rich volcanic clay from Java for this purpose. Here, the earth element, *ta-nah*, is prized for its ability to counter the effects of the sun and restore balance to body and mind. Mud from maritime regions, such as Dead Sea clay, is considered beneficial for its concentration of sea flora and fauna, containing vital trace elements taken up by the skin during use. The mint bath calls on the power of peppermint's ingredient menthol to cool irritated skin; the antiseptic herb also reduces body temperature by promoting perspiration, and the herby green bath bag contains bay leaves to soothe inflammation. The aloe vera gel in the massage blend is a surefire skin soother—research shows it to be a remarkable skin healer, used in hospitals to accelerate wound healing and treat burns. It is combined with lavender, the essential oil that encourages the growth of new skin cells. When, in the early years of the twentieth century, French chemist René Gattefossé rinsed a burn in lavender essence and noted the remarkably quick healing that followed, it led him to the study of plant essences, bringing about aromatherapy, the term he coined in 1937. Use once a week.

Caution: Avoid if you are pregnant or breast-feeding, have heart disease or high blood pressure; if you have sensitive skin, do a patch test for tea tree oil. Avoid sunlight and sunlamps for 6 hours after using the clay.

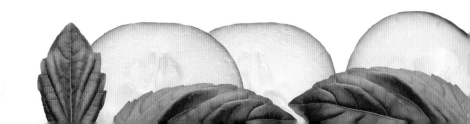

cooling clay mask (page 43)
1 cucumber, chilled and sliced thin

minty fresh bath bag (page 48)
cooling massage oil (page 15)

1 Warm the bathroom. Take handfuls of clay and smear it over the body, working methodically up from heels to shoulders. Make sure to cover all areas of redness.

2 Once covered in the aromatic clay, recline on an old towel for 15–20 minutes as the mask dries, placing a layer of overlapping cucumber slices over your face, eyes, and neck. Sip a glass of cool mineral water through a straw if desired.

3 Run a tepid bath, throwing in the mint bath bag. Remove the cucumber, shower off the clay with tepid water, then sink into the restorative herb bath.

4 After 10 minutes, climb out, pat dry gently, then massage all over with the cooling oil blend, working gently over skin that still feels delicate.

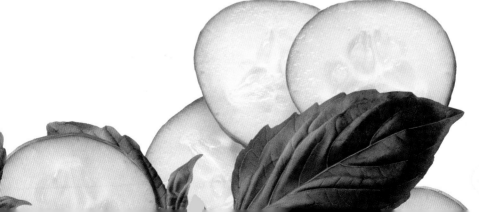

Warming steam treatment

A once-a-week sauna treatment for parched winter skin and hair, this home-spa treat is deep cleansing as well as moisturizing and very comforting on a frosty day. The heat of the steam causes blood vessels in the skin to dilate, increasing blood flow in the area and so boosting the interchange between waste products being expelled in perspiration and the uptake of nutrients in the steam. Apply the ylang ylang-scented hair mask before you subject yourself to the heat. Warmth boosts the moisturizing properties of this traditional tonic to stimulate hair growth and balance sebum in the scalp. Follow with a thorough body scrubbing Japanese style before stepping into a very hot bath for a few minutes. This is best done in the evening; very hot baths can drain you of energy and steam facials may leave the skin temporarily shiny and rather red. This is the perfect time to apply a night cream; heat-softened skin is especially receptive to deep moisturizing.

Caution: **Avoid if you are pregnant, have asthma or respiratory problems, high blood pressure, heart or vascular disease, or varicose veins; if you have sensitive skin, do a patch test for geranium and ylang ylang oils.**

You will need:

your regular skin cleanser
coconut hair-conditioning oil (page 14)
essential oil for your skin type:
lavender or jasmine for dry skin;
chamomile for sensitive skin; geranium
or sandalwood for normal skin;
lavender or patchouli for oily skin;
frankincense or rose for mature skin.

night cream of your choice
soap
wash mitt or loofah
shampoo and conditioner for your
   hair type
Eastern moisture balm (page 13)

1 Run a very hot bath, shutting doors and windows to keep the room steamy. Stand the bottle containing the coconut hair-conditioning oil in a bowl of hot water to warm. Cleanse your face in the usual way.

2 Slather hair in the warm coconut oil. Work through from roots to tips, massaging the head by moving the skin of the scalp firmly but gently with your fingertips as you work. Cover your hair and scalp with a plastic shower cap, then wrap in a warm towel.

3 Fill a bowl with 2 pints (1 liter) just-boiled water. Add 5 drops of one essential oil for your skin type. Cover your head with another towel and, keeping your face about 8 inches (24 cm) away from the water, eyes closed, cover your head and the bowl with a large towel to trap the steam. Remain under this tent for 5–10 minutes, breathing deeply. After emerging, place a cool, wet washcloth over your face and wipe away. Immediately moisturize using your favorite night cream.

4 In the shower (without getting your towel turban wet), briefly soak the body, then turn off the water and build up a lather of soap, scrubbing every inch with a hand mitt or wet loofah. Get squeaky clean.

5 Check the water temperature, then gingerly ease yourself into the very hot bath. Try to take it for as long as you can—up to 10 minutes for maximum benefits.

6 Rinse your hair in the shower, then shampoo and condition as usual.

7 Rub dry with a thick towel, then massage in the Eastern moisture oil, paying special attention to any areas of dry skin. Lie down with a glass of cool mineral water.

8 Now would be a good time to give yourself (or even better, get someone to give you) a pedicure or manicure (pages 72–74) while nails are softened. Alternatively, put on crisp clean pajamas and retire to bed for a good night's sleep.

87 Hammam steam soaping

Turkish baths, or *hammams*, are famous for their eucalyptus-scented steamy rooms. Less hot and more humid than a sauna, they guarantee a purifying sweat after around 10 minutes. In a hammam you relax on a heated marble slab, then submit to a vigorous massage using soapy suds and a gritty bath mitt before being sloshed with water and massaged with oil. Afterward skin is pink, fresh, and squeaky clean. If you can't find a Turkish bath near you, try this in your own bathroom. The eucalyptus oil clears the head while promoting concentration and alertness. The heat helps it to relieve aching muscles, deodorize the body, and clarify congested skin. The Turkish massage oil blend seeks to replicate the refreshing lemon cologne so popular across the country to refresh travelers and welcome guests. Use once a week.

Caution: Avoid during pregnancy and if you have high blood pressure, heart or vascular disease, or varicose veins; if you have epilepsy, omit eucalyptus oil.

You will need:

room vaporizer and 4 drops essential oil of eucalyptus	textured wash mitt
lemon-scented soap	Turkish massage blend (page 15)

1 Heat the bathroom until steamy by closing windows and doors and running a dangerously hot bath (do not get into it). To increase the steam further, place two large pans of just-boiled water on the floor in a corner where you are unlikely to upset them.

2 Place 4 drops of eucalyptus oil in water in the bowl of the vaporizer. Breathe in the piercing cool fumes, allowing them to clear congestion. This is especially effective if you have blocked sinuses, a runny nose, a cough, or a sore throat.

3 Take a warm shower but do not wash. While your skin is still wet, lather up the soap and massage the soft suds up over one arm and shoulder. Vigorously stroke up the whole arm, from wrist to shoulder, with the "V" of your working hand (between thumb and index finger). Glide back down and repeat, soaping gently over the top of the chest. Then knead around the back of the upper arm and shoulder, and up the side of the neck.

4 Using the mitt, scrub up the arm and around the shoulder making brisk up and down scrubbing actions. Work over as much of the top of the back as you can reach.

5 Repeat the massage from steps 3 and 4 on the other arm and shoulder. Then, work up another soapy lather, and massage up one leg from heel to thigh using large vigorous strokes, again creating lots of suds.

6 Using the "V" of one hand, then the other, push the flesh from above the knee up to the upper thigh, reaching around to work on as much of the leg as you can. Knead the inner and outer thigh and buttocks, passing the soapy flesh from one hand to another.

7 Using the mitt, scrub your heels, calves, thighs, and buttocks using the same zigzagging rubbing action as on the arms. Imagine erasing cellulite and flabby skin. Repeat on the other leg.

8 Work up yet more lather and massage your abdomen using circular strokes with the flat of both palms. Then work on one side of the abdomen, picking up handfuls of flesh with the "V" of one hand and passing them into the other hand. Knead in this way up from hips to ribs. Repeat on the other side, then scrub using the mitt as before, making small circular movements over the abdomen.

9 Take another shower, sloshing off the soap suds with warm water.

10 Rub vigorously with a thick towel, then massage still-moist skin all over with the Turkish massage oil blend.

88 Winter healing bath

Bathe away winter coughs and colds in a soothing bath. This balneary cold cure is a union of comforting and heating elements, with ginger at its center. Ginger has been considered a panacea across Asia, and particularly in Indonesia's herbal healing tradition, Jamu. It stimulates the circulatory system, is able to inhibit coughing, can relieve inflammation, and by increasing sweating helps reduce your body temperature if you have a fever. It also makes for a very aromatic bath. Essential oil of eucalyptus is skin stimulating, spirit livening, and penetrates a stuffy nose. The bath is preceded by body brushing—brisk, dry friction that stimulates the skin and lymphatic system and increases blood circulation. There is also a mini acupressure massage to help you breathe more easily while you wallow in the healing waters. Use once a week.

Caution: Avoid very hot baths during pregnancy and if you have high blood pressure, heart or vascular disease, or varicose veins; omit eucalyptus oil if you have epilepsy.

You will need:

4-in (10-cm) piece fresh ginger root	5 drops essential oil of eucalyptus
1 tsp honey	body brush
1 lemon	

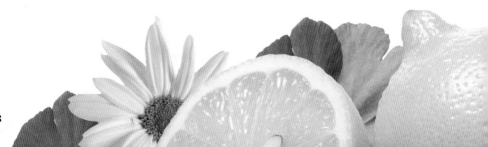

1 Grate one tablespoon of the ginger root into a cup. Pour over boiling water and allow to steep for 10 minutes. Sweeten with honey and, for extra anti-cold action, add a squeeze of fresh lemon juice.

2 Turn on the faucet to run a hot bath. Grate the remaining ginger root and throw into the bath as the water runs. (When emptying the bath, place a strainer over the drain.)

3 Dry-brush your skin with the body brush, using quick back-and-forth strokes up the body from the soles of the feet to the top of the shoulders. Be gentle over delicate areas such as the breasts. If you have no body brush, create the same effect by rubbing vigorously with a dry, non-fluffy towel.

4 Just before stepping into the bath, drop in the essential oil and swish with your fingers to disperse.

5 Relax in the bath, sipping the ginger tea, for up to 10 minutes. Feel cooling perspiration break out on your brow.

6 Between sips of your ginger tea, try a sinus-clearing acupressure mini-massage. Find the point on each side of your face about midway across the cheekbone, directly beneath the iris. Use the tips of your middle fingers to gently exert pressure on this point, hold for a moment, then release. Repeat the pressure several times.

7 Sit up slowly and step out of the bath carefully to prevent dizziness. Pat dry then wrap yourself in a comforting robe, drink a glass of cool mineral water, and lie down for 20 minutes.

89 Mocha moisture shower

As well as providing pep and zing for the central nervous system, fresh coffee beans make a great exfoliant for the skin. When fragranced with essential oil of cardamom (the pods are a traditional addition to coffee across the Arab world), the body blend becomes still more invigorating and awakening. Follow the coffee exfoliation with a coating of cocoa butter body lotion for its creamy sensuousness. Both coffee and cocoa contain properties that help protect the body from free radicals. These potentially cell-damaging molecules accumulate in reaction to overexposure to UV rays, pollution, cigarette smoke, and stress, and are thought to be implicated in 80 percent of skin-aging. The carrot rub also has powerful antioxidant effects: it is used in some Southeast Asian spas to bring nutrients to freshly exfoliated skin, including potassium and the antioxidant carotenoid beta-carotene that can convert into vitamin A for healthy skin and a boosted immune system. Use once a week for luminescent skin that's soft to the touch.

Caution: Avoid during pregnancy; if you have sensitive skin, do a patch test for cardamom oil.

You will need:

masculine coffee scrub (page 33)
loofah
2 large carrots, grated
cocoa butter body lotion of your choice

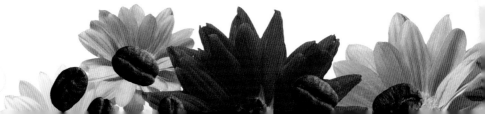

1 Brew yourself an espresso using freshly ground coffee beans. Enjoy the boosted alertness and concentration it brings. When the coffee grounds have cooled, but are still warm, remove them from the coffeemaker and use them to mix up the scrub, as described on page 33.

2 In a heated bathroom, rub handfuls of the coffee scrub from top to toe, taking 20 minutes or so to complete the treatment. Start at your feet and work up the body to your shoulders, making small circular strokes always in the direction of the heart, and using vigorous up and down scrubbing movements over areas of cellulite and rough skin. To increase the stimulation, once you are covered in the scrub, rub all over with a dampened loofah, focusing attention on your back and dry skin on your feet.

3 Shower away the scrub (place a strainer over the drain), savoring your silky skin with its sheen of oil. Don't use soap.

4 Now soothe your skin with handfuls of grated carrot, using expansive strokes to massage it all over your exfoliated skin. Focus on more sensitive areas, such as the chest and shins.

5 Shower away the grated carrot (ensuring the strainer is still in place over the drain), and pat dry.

6 Onto still-damp skin, massage copious amounts of cocoa butter body lotion. Then swaddle yourself in a cashmere blanket, and recline with a tall milky café latte, a glass of cooled mineral water, and a good book.

90   Tropical coconut bath

In spas across Thailand and Indonesia, a moisturizing coconut milk bath often follows skin-polishing exfoliation treatments. Here, the body scrub is a Balinese fresh coconut concoction: you rub handfuls of freshly grated coconut over the skin gently to remove dead cells and leave it glowing; it's good for sun-scorched skin, too. Then sink into a coconut bath scented with the aromas of Thailand, including lime and the essential oils of two grasses, lemongrass and vetivert. As you relax in the bath, give your hair a restoration treatment with a coconut conditioning oil containing essential oil of ylang ylang, distilled from flowers of a plant known as "the perfume tree" for their tenaciously heady scent. Ylang ylang was traditionally combined with coconut oil to create a hair serum by women in the South Seas, and it became the defining ingredient in nineteenth-century European Macasser hair oils. No wonder the tree was also named "crown of the East." Follow with a fresh lime hair rinse to reduce daily buildup of hair products and restore shine. Repeat every 2 weeks.

Caution: Avoid during pregnancy; if you have sensitive skin, do a patch test for ylang ylang oil.

You will need:

Balinese coconut-turmeric scrub (page 36)	lime hair tonic (page 49)
coconut hair-conditioning oil (page 14)	coconut milk bath (page 18)
shampoo for your hair type	conditioner for your hair type
	3 tbsp sweet almond oil
	2 tsp coconut oil

1 Heat the bathroom. Shower, then roughly dry your skin with a warm towel.

2 Take handfuls of the coconut scrub and rub into your still damp skin, working up from heels to shoulders. Start with long, broad strokes of the palms, sweeping toward the heart, then make small clockwise circles with your fingertips for an exfoliating effect. Pay special attention to areas of rough, dry skin, using a scrubbing action over your heels, knees, and elbows.

3 Relax for 20 minutes, sitting on an old towel, as you allow the coconut scrub to dry like a body mask. Spend the time applying the coconut conditioning oil to your scalp. Warm a little of the oil between your palms and rest them on the sides of your head, just behind the temples. Rotate your hands slowly, moving the skin, not just the hair. Place your fingertips at your hairline and make small circular pressures to rotate the skin of the scalp. Repeat, moving back over the head and down toward the nape of the neck.

4 Using a little more oil, place your fingertips on the top of your head and make zigzag movements down through the hair with your fingers. Finally, place your knuckles at the base of the skull and rotate them, moving over the head and neck wherever you still find pockets of tension. Close your eyes and relax for 5 minutes.

5 Shower off the coconut body mask and hair oil (place a strainer over the drain). Shampoo your hair and at the final rinse use the lime hair tonic, as directed on page 49.

6 Run a warm bath, adding the coconut milk ingredients. Sink in. Apply your favorite hair conditioner, gently moving the scalp with your fingertips as you work it through from roots to tips. Relax for 5 minutes, then shower off.

7 Pat dry with a warm towel. Blend the sweet almond and coconut oils then massage all over.

91 Thai spa ritual

Beauty treatments in Thai spas invariably include an acupressure foot massage. The bathing ritual that follows begins with a foot bath before progressing to an energizing foot massage, and also includes an invigorating and aromatic exfoliating body scrub scented with lemongrass. The scent of this grass permeates many Thai body treatments; it's almost as ubiquitous in these preparations as it is in the cuisine of the region, and is often picked fresh from the gardens of spa resorts for both dining and massage tables. As you might expect from its sharp lemony scent, essential oil distilled from the grass stems has an enlivening effect on the senses and body, lifting exhaustion, building an appetite, relieving the muscles of aches and pains (especially after a workout), and clearing the head. Beauticians value lemongrass for shrinking loose skin after weight loss or pregnancy, for toning open pores, and clarifying oily skin on the back. Use once a week.

Caution: Avoid during pregnancy; omit the bath bag if allergic to dairy products; if you have sensitive skin, do a patch test for lemongrass oil.

You will need:

mint tonic foot soak (page 49)	lemongrass milk bath bag (page 21)
Thai poppy seed scrub (page 37)	1 lime
loofah	lemon-scented body lotion of your choice

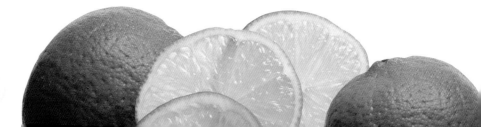

1 Heat the bathroom. Add the mint infusion to a bucket of warm water. Sit on a chair with the bucket in front of you and soak your feet and calves in the refreshing water for five minutes. Step out and pat dry.

2 Massage your body with handfuls of the aromatic scrub, working up from calves to shoulders. Then rub all over briskly with a dampened loofah, making circular strokes always in the direction of the heart. Wash your hands.

3 Relax for 20 minutes. Cover a chair with an old towel and sit down to give yourself an acupressure foot treatment. Place one foot on your opposite thigh; try not to cover it in the scrub. Sandwich the foot between your hands. Rotate at the ankle, moving the foot clockwise and counterclockwise several times.

4 Sandwiching the toes between your hands, flex them toward the shin, then point them downward several times. Briskly rub the foot between your palms to warm it.

5 Apply pressure with your thumb along the arch of the foot, working from heel to big toe: depress, hold, circle, then release, moving along a little to repeat the action.

6 Exert pressure all around the ball of the foot, beneath the big toe, working carefully into areas that feel tense or tender.

7 Now make pressures in the same way around the ankle, especially beneath the ankle bone. Finish with more soothing sandwiching strokes along the length of the foot. Repeat on the other foot.

8 Shower away the body scrub (place a strainer over the drain).

9 Run a warm bath, throwing in the lemongrass bath bag as the water runs. Relax in the softening herbal bath for 10 minutes. Sip a glass of mineral water with a squeeze of lime juice.

10 Pat dry, then rehydrate the skin with a lemony scented body lotion.

Balinese spice treatment

After a long day in the paddy fields, Balinese workers would use this rub of crushed spices known as *boreh* to relieve aching joints and overworked muscles, and warm the body, especially during the cold, rainy season. Now an adaptation of the treatment is a mainstay of spas worldwide. This stimulating treat is not for the faint hearted (it's spicily warm on the skin), but its circulation-boosting properties are recommended by spa therapists for clients suffering from tired aching muscles, for fitness fanatics who have overdone the training, and to counter jet lag. While the body scrub dries, try a ginger-infused foot massage oil that has analgesic properties, stimulates circulation to the extremities, helps heal blisters, and relieves cramps and strains after a long day standing or walking. The oil blend is said to be very grounding, which makes it even more appropriate for the feet. This muscle-relaxant treatment is best carried out in the evening. Use once a week.

Caution: Avoid if you are pregnant or have very sensitive skin.

You will need:

1 in (2.5 cm) piece fresh ginger root	Malay spice bath oil (page 12)
1–2 tsp honey	*boreh* body rub (page 34)
lemon and ginger foot massage oil (page 15)	exotic body lotion of your choice

1 Heat the bathroom and run a warm bath. Finely grate the ginger root into a cup and pour just-boiled water over it. Allow to steep for 10 minutes, then sweeten with honey. Make up the foot massage oil in a bottle and place the bottle to warm in a bowl of hot water. Before stepping into the bath, pour the Malay spice oil into the water, swishing with your fingers to disperse the oils.

2 Relax in the water for 10 minutes, sipping the ginger tea. Try to let go of muscular tension: imagine exhaling aches and pains as you breathe out. As you start to perspire visualize toxins exiting your skin.

3 Step out of the bath and towel dry. To still-damp skin, apply the boreh rub, massaging handfuls up from your ankles to the tops of your shoulders. Use small circular strokes, rubbing in a clockwise direction and always working toward the heart. Appreciate the warmth acting on aching muscles.

4 Allow the rub to dry on your skin for 10 minutes. Sit on a chair covered with a large old towel and, while you're waiting, ease aching feet further with a ginger-infused massage.

5 Bend one leg and place the foot on your opposite thigh. Try not to cover it in the rub. Pour a little of the massage oil into one palm and rub both palms together. Warm the foot by sandwiching it between your palms and sweeping down from ankle to toes several times.

6 Inch up the sole, from heel to toes, walking alternate thumbs like a caterpillar. Start at the instep, repeat down the center of the sole, then on the outer edge.

7 Run your thumb along the grooves on the top of the foot leading between each toe, working from the base of the toe toward the shin.

8 Massage each toe between your thumb and index finger, rotating and rubbing from base to tip and pressing firmly at the tip before pulling away.

9 Ripple your knuckles all over the sole to finish. Repeat on the other foot.

10 Shower off the spice treatment, placing a strainer over the drain to catch any debris.

11 Pat dry and to still-damp skin apply an exotic body lotion—look for one containing extracts of ginger, jasmine, and ylang ylang. Put on a luxurious robe and drink a glass of refreshing mineral water.

Breton thalassotherapy treatment

In France the art of harnessing the benefits of the marine environment—its climate and salt water, waves and seaweed, mud and sand—has been refined in *thalassotherapie* (*thalassa* means sea in Greek). The first sea treatment institute opened in 1899 and there are now around 40 establishments, especially in the Brittany region, where 90 percent of seaweed used in Europe is harvested. At a thalassotherapy spa you bathe in heated seawater piped directly from the ocean, are pummeled with jets of water, enveloped in seaweed, and massaged with extracts of marine algae. Seaweed has impressive skincare claims made for it: the iodine content is reputed to ward off signs of aging and repair the effects of sun damage, while its high mineral content (different varieties contain differing amounts of sodium, calcium, potassium, iron, copper, magnesium, and zinc) is said by thalassotherapists to impart a smoothing and firming mini-lift; nutrients stimulate the fibroblast cells that produce collagen for a skin-plumping effect. Certainly, seaweed treatments leave skin looking and feeling soft and refreshed. Salt and seaweed baths promote perspiration for a detoxifying action. When the water is heated to 93.2–98.6°F (34–37°C), vasodilation takes place in the dermal tissues, allowing the mineral contents of the bathwater to penetrate the skin. The temperature is thought to account also for the boosted blood circulation, relieved cramps and muscle tension claimed for the therapy. To replicate the effects at home, seek out *sel gris* from Guérande in Brittany or *sel aux alguës* containing flecks of seaweed. The relaxing body-temperature bath is followed by a bracing shower that stimulates areas of cellulite with water jets, as do the stern therapists in thalassotherapy spas who target problem areas with hydro-therapy. Use once a week.

Caution: Avoid if you are pregnant or have high blood pressure or heart disease, if you are allergic to iodine or seafood, or if you are taking thyroxine; omit essential oil of juniper if you have kidney disease, rosemary if you have high blood pressure or epilepsy.

You will need:

silky sea salt scrub (page 27), substituting the 4 drops essential oil of peppermint with 4 drops each cypress and lavender and 2 drops juniper

seaweed salt soak (page 25)
anticellulite massage blend (page 15)

1 Run a warm bath, measuring the temperature with a thermometer until it reaches 93.2–98.6°F (34–37°C).

2 While the bath is running, take handfuls of the sea salt scrub and massage from heels to shoulders using firm circular strokes, always working in the direction of the heart. Pay close attention to areas of cellulite—rough, dimpled skin around the thighs, buttocks, abdomen, and upper arms.

3 Add the seaweed solution to the bath and swish to disperse before stepping in. Relax for 12 minutes, thought to be the optimum time for penetration of trace elements and minerals in the salt water. You might like to put on a CD of sea sounds, close your eyes, and visualize a seascape or a tropical beach. Breathe out tension with every exhalation, and inhale the calming scents of the sea. Keep a glass of cool mineral water on hand to rehydrate you as you perspire.

4 Step into the shower and rinse away the salt and seaweed extracts. Then, using the shower head, give yourself a bracing blast over areas of cellulite, moving the jet in small circles over the thighs, buttocks, and abdomen, making the water gradually as cool as you dare.

5 Rub dry vigorously with a thick towel.

6 Finish with an invigorating massage with the anticellulite oil blend. Use long, smooth strokes to cover the thighs, buttocks, and abdomen, then pummel and knead the flesh, giving it a good going over with the knuckles of both hands. Then use smooth, upward sculpting strokes from knee to hip to soothe and relax.

94   Javanese *Lulur* celebration

For at least 500 years, courtesans in Java's royal palaces have been bathed and pampered for 40 days before a wedding with *lulur*, a skin-softening blend of sweet and spicy powders impregnated with heavenly scented essential oils. The treatment was thought to prepare body and mind for the wedding night and even to aid conception. This beautifying treatment leaves skin silky soft, glowing, and perfumed, and like the Balinese *boreh* body rub (page 34), has been adopted enthusiastically by spas around the world. Jasmine, a key component of the powder, is well known as an aphrodisiac and is a star ingredient of love potions (the essential oil is reputed to boost a man's sperm count!). Applied to the skin, jasmine oil increases suppleness, especially for dry and sensitive complexions, while the sweetly sensual, almost overwhelming floral aroma seems to wipe away worries and induce positivity (something every bride could use in the month before her wedding). Use once a week.

Caution: Avoid if pregnant or allergic to dairy products.

You will need:

jasmine skincare oil (page 12)
lulur powder scrub (page 35)
large container live natural yogurt

handfuls of rose petals
jasmine tea bag
floral body lotion of your choice

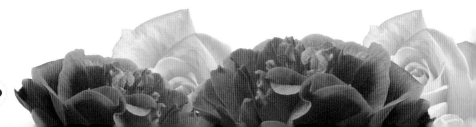

1 Make sure the bathroom is well heated. Massage every part of your body with the jasmine oil. Take time to reach all those hard-to-get-to areas, breathing in the heady scent.

2 Apply handfuls of the *lulur* scrub to your skin, massaging it in by making gentle circles with your fingertips. Start at your heels and work up to the top of your shoulders. Pay extra attention to patches of rough skin around the knees and elbows, heels and buttocks.

3 Relax for 10 minutes, sitting on an old towel, while the paste dries on your skin.

4 Using small circular fingertip strokes, rub off the paste, exfoliating the skin as you do so.

5 Splash handfuls of cool yogurt over your skin, covering the areas treated by the *lulur* scrub. Shower off.

6 Run a warm bath, scattering the rose petals over the water. Place the jasmine tea bag in a cup and pour over just-boiled water. Allow to steep for 5 minutes. Sink into the bath, luxuriating in the flower water for 20 minutes while you sip the jasmine tea.

7 Step out of the bath and pat skin dry with a warm fluffy towel. While your skin is still damp, apply a floral-scented body lotion—look for one containing extracts of jasmine, rose, or geranium.

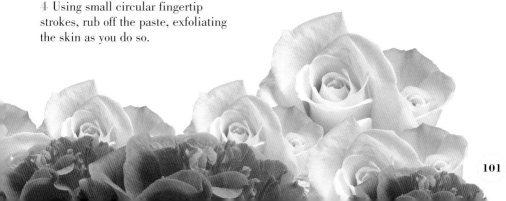

95 Indian oil bath

This fragrant prebath massage is inspired by a twelfth-century Indian text that outlines a daily bathing ritual of oiling and massage with scented ointments made up of jasmine, coriander, cardamom, basil, pine, saffron, and clove enwrapped in sesame oil. Oiling the body is said to draw toxins to the surface to be washed away, ensuring increased well-being and, Ayurvedic doctors claim, peace of mind. This blend of scented oils especially suits dry skin and complexions in need of renewal. It warms sore muscles and lifts exhaustion while refreshing the senses and reviving the mind. Bring your attention to each area of your body that your hands pass over, breathing new life into the area with every inhalation, and breathing out tension as you exhale. The oiling is followed by a saffron bath, once enjoyed by Roman emperors for its perfuming and aphrodisiac powers, and ability to raise the spirits. Make this bath a weekly treat.

Caution: Omit jasmine and basil oils during pregnancy; if you have sensitive skin, do a patch test for basil, pine, and cardamom oils.

You will need:

room vaporizer and 2 drops essential oil of clove	Indian body blend (page 14)
Indian face balm (page 14)	saffron infusion (page 48)

1 Heat the bathroom. Drop the clove oil into the water bowl of the room vaporizer. Pour a little of the face balm into one palm and rub between both palms to warm it. Rest the fingertips of both hands on your chin and stroke up your jawline, swiveling at the wrists to circle your middle fingers at the temples. Repeat.

2 Rest your fingertips on each side of your nose, and draw outward, again swiveling at the wrists to circle the temples with your fingers. Repeat. Then place your fingertips at the center of your forehead. Draw outward and circle at the temples. Repeat.

3 If you don't mind coating your hair with oil, warm a little more face balm between your palms and place your spread fingertips on your hairline, little fingers touching in the center, thumbs beside your ears. Circle the scalp, moving the skin against the skull. Move your fingers back an inch and repeat. Repeat up and over your head and down to the nape of your neck.

4 Pour a little of the body blend into one palm and rub between both palms to warm. Place your palms horizontally on your abdomen, one just above your navel, the other just below. Start to circle the palms clockwise, lifting one over the other as they meet.

5 Add a little more oil, then stroke up and over your chest (avoid the breasts) to circle opposite shoulders. Rub oil over as much of your back as you can

reach, squeezing the large muscles around your neck and shoulders.

6 Apply a little more oil and slide one palm up the opposite arm from wrist to shoulder. Circle the shoulder joint and glide back down to repeat. Briefly massage the hands, before working on the other arm in the same way.

7 Apply more oil, and, kneeling up, massage your buttocks robustly, pounding and kneading the flesh.

8 Using more oil, massage the thigh, calf, and sole of one leg and foot, circling the hip, knee, and ankle. Keep the strokes flowing and knead into fleshy areas. Devote time to each toe, pulling away at the tip. Repeat on the other leg and foot.

9 Relax for 5 minutes lying on your back on an old towel while the oil absorbs. Run a warm bath, adding the saffron infusion just before stepping in. Relax for 20 minutes. Don't wash off all the oil—allow a little to remain on the skin to nourish and hydrate it.

96 May day love bath

Across Europe, May Day is a traditional time for beautifying rituals and outdoor courtship festivals that mark the start of the summer. In the past celebrations would begin at dawn with a dewdrop face bath. Bathing in the dew on this day of the year is considered particularly good for the complexion, with the power to guard against the aging effects of exposure to the sun and lessen the appearance of freckles. Some traditions claim the effects will last all year. Others say you will marry the first man you meet after washing with the dew. This was the inspiration for this flight of fancy bathing ritual for single women in search of Mr. Right. It includes a love potion to stir into the water in hopeful anticipation, and a wish, all the more powerful if made before sunrise. The floral water is an instant *eau de cologne* or "miracle water," essential to the bathing rituals of sixteenth-century Europe, when the mix of herbs, spices, and natural essences was a secret closely guarded by the monks and nuns who created many of them. Take this bath in the morning, then think of yourself as your very own queen of the May for the day.

You will need:

flower water skin splash (page 49)
handfuls of fresh rose petals and
lavender flowers

lavender pillow

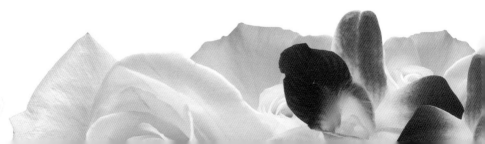

1 Before going to bed on the last day of April, creep outdoors and hang a washcloth on the clothesline. When you wake early on May Day morning, venture outside and before doing anything else, wash your face in the dew gathered on the washcloth. As you do so, make a wish to meet "The One" this spring.

2 Go a-Maying today: take a walk in the countryside or woodland to gather boughs of young green-leafed trees and blossom to decorate the home. Do not gather hawthorn, otherwise known as May blossoms, which is considered unlucky if brought indoors.

3 Fill your bathroom with fresh seasonal flowers: pots of lilac, crinkly tulips and scented narcissi, boughs of cherry and apple blossom, lily of the valley in cut-glass, and jelly jars of the first clove-scented pinks.

4 Run a bath as you mix up the flower water. Think of it as a love potion. As you drop in the essential oils, stir them with a swizzle stick, writing the initials of your loved one's name. Visualize his face appearing in the water, and imagine what your opening line to him might be.

5 Cast the rose petals and lavender flowers into the water, then step into the bath, resting your head on a lavender pillow, if possible. Close your eyes and imagine all the possibilities for love awaiting you. Make a decision to put yourself into all kinds of new situations, and to stay open to whatever fate may bring.

6 Step out of the bath, pat dry with a luxuriously huge towel, splash yourself with the light floral body water, dress in your finery, then go out for the day.

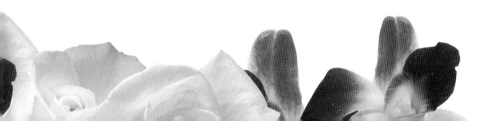

97   Girly fairy bath

For girly girls of any age, 3 to 33, here is a magical pink bath to make your dreams come true. Enjoy in the early evening when, lit with candles, the bubbles glitter. Pink baths call on the softest hues of the red spectrum, which in color healing therapy are recommended to promote love and kindness. For small girls, search party stores for tiny plastic fairies for make-believe bath games—play hide-and-seek in the bubbles. For grown-ups, augment the feelings of love pink is thought to promote with a little essential oil of rose, which lifts the spirits, washes away everyday stress, and boosts femininity. Buy the best quality you can afford. Complete the bath by coating skin with a sheen of glittery body lotion for dazzling shine and sparkle, or a shake of fairy dust.

Caution: Avoid rose oil during pregnancy.

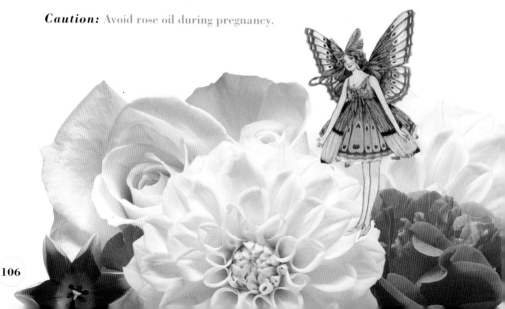

You will need:

candles in shades of pink and lilac
glittery bath bubbles (page 29)
essential oil of rose, optional

glitter body lotion of your choice
vanilla dusting powder (fairy dust)
(page 31)

1 Fill the room with candles, votives, and nightlights (for children's baths, make sure they're out of reach of small hands).

2 Run a warm bath, adding the glitter bubble solution beneath the faucet. Marvel as the tub fills with pink glittery bubbles.

3 Just before stepping in, swish in 10 drops essential oil of rose if you are over the age of 18. As you step into the bath, the oil on the surface will coat your skin with its aphrodisiac, antidepressant, and pleasantly sedative properties.

4 Relax in the bath for 20 minutes or so. Ponder which kind of fairy you'd like to be—queen of the fairies or a fairy godmother; a good fairy perhaps, or do bad fairies have more fun? Conjure up three wishes, then make them, washing in an upward direction as you do so to bring in good luck.

5 Step out of the bath and pat dry with a warm fluffy towel. Apply a glittery body lotion or, once dry, sprinkle yourself with the fairy dust. Put on your favorite fairy dress, be it a frilly tulle tutu or a gossamer-like wisp of scarlet silk. Add wings and a wand and you're ready to make magic.

98 Crackling champagne bath

An exciting bath for adults only, accompanied by a flute of chilled champagne. This effervescent experience is the ideal pep-me-up after a long day at work when you have a big night ahead. It contains stimulating ginger to zing up the senses, lift tiredness and a bad mood, and relieve weary muscles of their stresses and strains. The bathwater has best effects at body temperature, which might feel a little cool when you first climb in. Be wary of using too-hot water for an evening bath when you need to go out—it can make you feel sleepy and drain the will to socialize. At the end of this bath, run in a little extra cool water for instant invigoration. Follow with a moisturizing massage using an invigorating body oil. Its spicy fragrance, composed of coriander and cardamom oils, is thought to remove any remaining lethargy by refreshing and inspiring. Ancient Egyptians regarded coriander as the spice of happiness, perhaps because of its uplifting effect on the nervous system and aphrodisiac reputation. If this doesn't get the party started, nothing will.

Caution: Avoid while pregnant or breast-feeding; if you have sensitive skin, do a patch test for cardamom, pine, basil, and ginger oils.

You will need:

crackling bath crystals (page 30) | oatmeal skin scrub bag (page 47)
bottle of champagne | Indian body blend (page 14)

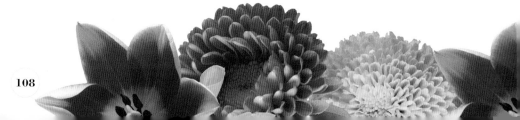

1 Run a tepid bath. Put on your favorite, lively "going out" music. "I'm Coming Out" by Diana Ross is always a good choice. Open the champagne, and pour a glass into a chilled champagne flute. Refrigerate the bottle.

2 Mix up the bath crystals, keeping them dry until you sprinkle them over the water just before stepping in. Breathe in the awakening scents and let the snap, crackle, and pop remind you of the wakefulness of breakfast time.

3 Relax in the bath, sipping the champagne. Let it go to your head, relishing the rush the bubbles bring, and anticipating the evening's entertainment. Don't be tempted to climb out to pour one more glass— you might never get out of the house!

4 Scrub all over with the rose and oatmeal bath bag. Let the oatmeal fill the bath with its soothing milky solution.

5 Just before you're ready to emerge, turn on the cold faucet and run in a little cool water, swishing it with your hands like paddles so the invigorating waves circulate around you. When you feel full of get-up-and-go, get out of the bath.

6 Dry yourself with a vigorous rub of a thick towel.

7 Massage all over with the vivifying Indian body oil, making sure to warm the large muscles in the arms and legs with stimulating circular strokes toward the heart. Wait for 15 minutes or so for the oil to be absorbed by your skin before getting dressed to avoid getting oil stains on your party finery.

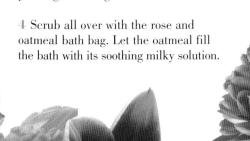

99   Sensuous candlelight bath

Most warm baths have an aphrodisiac effect, soothing away physical aches and pains, helping the mind give up worries, and focusing attention on the pleasures of the body. This aphrodisiac bath strewn with rose petals employs the love-inducing qualities of essential oils used for wedding baths across the world. As well as coating the skin with a luxuriously scented sheen that makes it irresistible for touching, the bath oil contains the famed aphrodisiac oils jasmine, sandalwood, and patchouli; all have played a role since ancient times in seduction and lovemaking. With its penetrating earthy aroma, patchouli is a famed aphrodisiac that is also used to regenerate the skin and treat cellulite. Jasmine, another skin-softening oil, adds an intense floral note to the mix, and is said to be particularly good for male sexual problems. The lingering-scented sandalwood wipes away anxiety and relaxes women in particular. Start with a skin-softening fruity body treatment that makes you feel good enough to eat. Use once a week.

Caution: Omit essential oil of jasmine during pregnancy; avoid the body mask if you are allergic to dairy products.

You will need:

candles	Eastern moisture balm (page 13)
patchouli incense (optional)	handfuls of rose petals, fresh or dried
banana body moisture mask (page 43)	jasmine-scented soap

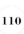

1 Heat the bathroom and run a warm, deep bath. Light candles and a stick or cone of patchouli incense, if you (and your lover) appreciate its intense fragrance. While the water is running, mix up the banana body mask and picking up handfuls, rub it all over the skin, starting at your heels and working up the body to your shoulders. Make circular motions with your fingertips, scrubbing at areas of hard skin and soothing hardened muscles with smooth strokes. Relax for 20 minutes lying on an old towel as the mask dries.

2 Stand under a warm shower and rinse away the mask (place a strainer over the drain to catch the organic matter). Enjoy the sensation of fresh rivulets of water cascading over your freshly deep-cleansed skin. Imagine yourself showering outdoors beneath a tropical waterfall.

3 Pour a little of the Eastern moisture balm into the filled bath, swishing to disperse into a film on the surface of the water. Throw in the rose petals (place a strainer over the drain when emptying the bath to catch them).

4 Step into the water, allowing the oil film to coat your body. Relax here for 20 minutes or more. Relive your favorite romantic encounters in your imagination while you soak. Wash with the jasmine-scented soap.

5 Step out of the bath, patting your body dry with a soft, warm towel carefully, so as not to rub away the oils on the surface of the skin. Don a fresh robe and retire to your boudoir.

6 Use the remaining Eastern moisture balm for sensual massage.

Resources

CHOCOLATE BATH PRODUCTS
www.Serendipity3.com Serendipity restaurant and general store for chocolate bath and skincare lines.
225 East 60th Street,
New York, NY 10022
Tel: (212) 838-3531

www.rubber-ducky.com great natural bath products, including chocolate treats, shipped to homes in the U.S.

COLOR BATH PRODUCTS
www.equinoxbooksandgifts.com for all-natural color bath sachets of every hue.

FAIRY BATH PRODUCTS
www.efairies.com the online fairy store for everything from fairy dust and wings to bath time lotions and potions.

HAMMAM ACCESSORIES
www.HasanSoyer.com for various Turkish bath sets, bowls, clogs, hand mitts, pumice stones, natural soaps, loofahs, and towels.

INDONESIAN BOREH AND JAMU PRODUCTS
www.jamuspa.com for home spa kits and products, including boreh body scrubs that are inspired by Indonesian Jamu healthcare.

JAPANESE BATH PRODUCTS
www.naturaljapanesebeauty.com for salts blended to replicate the waters at Kusatu, Hakone, Shirahama, and Shirabone resorts.

www.itmonline.org for Meito umi onsen, outdoor spring, salts.

www.fastriver.com/onsen Canadian online onsen guide selling Tabi no yado, or "Traveller's Inn," bath powders.

WINE SPA PRODUCTS
www.caudalie.com products for skin and baths from extracts of grapes developed by Mathilde Cathiard from the Chateau Smith Haut Lafitte wine estate with dermatologists from Bordeaux University.